CONTEMPORARY COMMUNITY HEALTH SERIES

Titles in the Series

ANATOMY OF A COORDINATING COUNCIL
Implications for Planning
Basil J. F. Mott

BRITISH PRIVATE MEDICAL PRACTICE
AND THE NATIONAL HEALTH SERVICE
Samuel Mencher

CHILDREN IN JEOPARDY
A Study of Abused Minors and Their Families
Elizabeth Elmer

DENTISTS, PATIENTS, AND AUXILIARIES
Margaret Cussler and Evelyn W. Gordon

DYNAMICS OF INSTITUTIONAL CHANGE
The Hospital in Transition
Milton Greenblatt, Myron R. Sharaf, and Evelyn M. Stone

EDUCATION AND MANPOWER FOR COMMUNITY HEALTH
Hilary G. Fry, with William P. Shepard and Ray H. Elling

HOME TREATMENT
Spearhead of Community Psychiatry
Leonard Weiner, Alvin Becker, and Tobias T. Friedman

MARRIAGE AND MENTAL HANDICAP
Janet Mattinson

METHODOLOGY IN EVALUATING
THE QUALITY OF MEDICAL CARE
An Annotated Selected Bibliography, 1955–1968
Isidore Altman, Alice J. Anderson, and Kathleen Barker

MIGRANTS AND MALARIA IN AFRICA
R. Mansell Prothero

A PSYCHIATRIC RECORD MANUAL FOR THE HOSPITAL
Dorothy Smith Keller

DYNAMICS OF INSTITUTIONAL CHANGE

DYNAMICS
OF

Milton Greenblatt
Myron R. Sharaf
Evelyn M. Stone

University of Pittsburgh Press

INSTITUTIONAL CHANGE

The Hospital in Transition

Publication of this book was made possible by a grant from the Maurice Falk Medical Fund. The Fund, however, is not the author, publisher, or proprietor of the material presented here and is not to be understood, by virtue of its grant, as endorsing any statement made or expressed herein.

Library of Congress Catalog Card Number 79-139597
ISBN 0-8229-3222-9
Copyright © 1971, University of Pittsburgh Press
Henry M. Snyder & Co., Inc., London
Manufactured in the United States of America

Publication of this book
was made possible by a grant
from the Maurice Falk Medical Fund.

For Rog, Giselle, and Sam

Contents

Preface

This volume was initially stimulated by the senior author's experiences as superintendent of Boston State Hospital from the spring of 1963 to the summer of 1967. The varied challenges of administering and attempting to modify a large mental hospital—an organizational setting which has many parallels and similarities to other public institutions—over time came to demand close scrutiny. During these years, the superintendent joined forces with a social scientist (Myron R. Sharaf) and a communicator (Evelyn M. Stone), and together we began to take notes and to document some of the currents that were moving us along in the process of change.

However, it was not until the senior author left the hospital that there was the opportunity and detachment to pull our experiences together in a more systematic fashion. During the period of more precise formulation and writing, we became more convinced than ever that the leadership role in a large mental hospital, or for that matter in any human-service organization, should be made as much an object of study and investigation as specific therapeutic, educational, or rehabilitative modalities. We also became convinced that the administrative art is too often locked in the minds of men who have been through the mill, but who have not had the time or inclination to think conceptually about their problems, methods, and techniques. Too often, administration is still regarded as "dirty work," an unnecessary nuisance at best, instead of being seen as the matrix within which vigorous, positive developments are either nurtured or extinguished.

In the long chain of circumstances that led to the creation of this book, outstanding to the senior author was the opportunity to live and work in such an exciting and reactive organization as Massachusetts Mental Health Center. There, the leadership of two successive administrators, Harry C. Solomon and Jack R. Ewalt, helped to formulate his concept of the executive prototype, and the rapid changes from custodial to therapeutic care heightened his awareness of the significance of administrative functions, the forces relating to proper institutional management, and the dynamics of organizational change. In his dual role as director of a large research organization and as assistant superintendent, he was exposed to the many stimulating experiences and events that played a part in shaping his intellectual principles.

Most influential in advancing his sophistication in the socioenvironmental sphere during this period were: Esther Lucille Brown, Doris Gilbert, George Grosser, Richard Hodgson, Gerald Klerman, Bernard Kramer, David Landy, Daniel Levinson, Myron R. Sharaf, Henry Wechsler, Frederick Wells, Richard Williams, and Richard York.

Of those who contributed greatly to the successful changes at Boston State Hospital we count: Arnold Abrams, John Arsenian, Alvin Becker, Robert Caplan, Ching-Piao Chien, Melvin Cohen, Jerome Collins, Floyd Cross, Alberto DiMascio, Peter DiNatale, Frederick Duhl, Ann Evans, Michael Gill, Wilmot Griffith, Ernest Hartmann, David Kantor, Ernest Kraus, Anton Kris, Betty Glasser Lifson, Davide Limentani, Matthew Luzzi, Mabel McKenzie, Turner McLardy, John Moskovites, Michael Murphy, David Myerson, Anna Pandiscio, John Porter, Alan Rothstein, Lawrence Schiff, Theodore Schoenfeld, John Snell, Maida Solomon, Bernard Stotsky, Nicholas Thisse, and Leonard Weiner, among others.

For her infinite patience and invaluable editorial assistance in the preparation of this manuscript, we are indebted to Margaret Hamwey.

We are grateful to the Maurice Falk Medical Fund, whose generous endowment made this book possible. And for his personal involvement far beyond his function as president of that foundation, we owe our deep thanks to Philip B. Hallen.

The Authors

MILTON GREENBLATT, M. D., is commissioner of the Massachusetts Department of Mental Health, professor of psychiatry at Tufts University School of Medicine and lecturer in psychiatry at Harvard Medical School and the Boston University School of Medicine. He has published widely in the field of psychiatry.

MYRON R. SHARAF, Ph.D., is currently associate area director of Boston State Hospital and assistant professor of psychology at Tufts University School of Medicine. His articles on psychology, hospital administration, and community organization have appeared in many periodicals in the field.

EVELYN M. STONE serves as executive editor for the Massachusetts Department of Mental Health.

Prologue

Few social issues are more important today than the question of changing our public institutions so that they are more responsive to human want. Our cumulative knowledge of what people need far outstrips our current capacity to translate this information into concrete service for our citizenry. This problem is likely to become more severe as our population expands and as people become better informed, through broader education and mass media, of the gap between what *is* and what *should be.*

Our large, slow-moving, rigid bureaucracies threaten our social and moral commitments because they so often fail to act appropriately and swiftly to meet ongoing challenges. They also fail us badly because their inflexibility and obeisance to the dead hand of custom often make them unable to recruit as staff precisely those people most interested in working in the field of public service—the young and idealistic. Obviously, something needs to be done to make a better congruence among the clear-cut needs of the people, the institutions presumably devoted to meeting these needs, and the enthusiastic energies of those who are willing to work under difficult circumstances but who are unwilling to find their efforts atrophied by paralyzing rigidities.

This book is concerned with the transitional period in the reorganization of a large public institution. Its primary focus is on the problems hampering change and the gains and losses of one or another strategy of change. To use the language of research, we are more concerned with the study of process than with outcome.

Our case study is a large mental hospital, Boston State Hospital, where the senior author served as superintendent from the spring of 1963 to the summer of 1967. It is our hope that the concepts advanced herein will be applicable not only to mental institutions but to other human-service organizations as well, such as municipal hospitals, schools and colleges, welfare agencies, prisons, and the like. Although much of the material we draw on is perforce concerned with psychiatric services, this book is *not* primarily about psychiatry, but about the administrative issues involved in trying to make a complex public facility more alive, more flexible, and more responsive to the people it serves. It is self-evident that an organization cannot meet the needs of its clients unless it also meets many of the needs of its staff; much of our material, therefore, will deal with problems of staff morale, education, and collaboration.

The state hospital offers singular advantages as a case study for analyzing problems inherent in organizational change. Difficulties that many institutions face are particularly acute in publicly supported mental hospitals, which usually have a low staff-patient ratio, low staff morale, and less than optimum patient care. They absorb a large share of the state budget but are rarely anything the state points to as one of its major accomplishments. They are often isolated from the community, not always because of distance alone, although many are in rural areas to "protect the public from the inmates." More significantly, they have been isolated because the public fears mental illness and because hospital personnel have developed, like members of other bureaucracies, ingrown, defensive attitudes that make them want to eschew close public contact and the scrutiny of reformers.

Our story describes our attempt to alter the organization of one such large institution to make it more responsive to the needs of patients, staff, and community. Both in the course of administrative practice and in our present effort to look back and understand what happened, we have made considerable use of the concepts of social science. This text in part reflects the marriage between social science and psychiatry, a relationship which has had its ups and downs but which has endured and still remains a vigorous one.

We cannot here give any extensive bibliography of the literature on this subject, but we do wish to mention some of the works that have been most influential in formulating our own philosophy of administration. These include Maxwell Jones's seminal description of the therapeutic community[1] and Stanton and Schwartz's richly detailed account of organizational life and its effect on patients in a private psychiatric institution.[2] Both these books opened up new avenues of exploration in social psychiatry. They stimulated or planted the novel idea that psychiatric administration is not simply a necessary evil but could be vitally important in setting the conditions for successful treatment of patients. Moreover, they and the books and articles of others, such as Caudill,[3] Wilmer,[4] Bellak,[5] and Linn,[6] demonstrated that administrative psychiatry also constituted a fascinating area for the conceptual study of the interplay between intrapsychic and social factors.

These studies sometimes implicitly called attention to the role of top leadership in developing more therapeutic administrative practice. More systematic, detailed studies of the leadership process have been few. We would, however, call attention to one unusual effort by Hodgson, Levinson, and Zaleznik[7] to unravel the significance of the executive role constellation of three top leaders of a small mental hospital. The authors revealed the relationship between role and personality, the pattern of communication, and the partition of power and function within the leadership triangle.

Our study will also concentrate heavily on questions of leadership. It is clear that if change, and fairly rapid change, is to occur in our large organizations, considerable impetus must come from the top. But guidelines for the administrator trying to institute change are rare, as rare as training programs to prepare him for this kind of organizational challenge.

Taking psychiatry as an example, young men with minimum field experience or technical skill have been catapulted into positions of great administrative responsibility. Their training has often been concentrated on their role as therapist; that is, they have learned how to deal with an individual patient or small groups of patients, but generally they have not been trained as administrators. If they were lucky, they may at least have had the experience of running a ward or had been apprenticed to a senior tutor with some skill in organizational matters. Some young men from university settings have been double-jumped into highly responsible positions without even the opportunity to try their wings at leading an organization of any size whatsoever.

The lack of training programs in administration is one reason for the present leadership gap in psychiatry—the many open executive positions and the relatively few candidates for them. Another reason is that many psychiatrists are just not interested in executive posts, particularly in a large state institution. One can well understand why. Their background in medicine, with its high value on the direct doctor-patient relationship, the fascination of dealing with individual psychopathology, and many other personal factors lead these young men mostly to clinical practice. Why take on a high administrative position in a public institution? Why expose oneself to unnecessary hardships, political pressures, goldfish-bowl scrutiny, criticisms, accusations, and possible public investigations?

Indeed, top executive jobs in many of our public institutions are not for those who dislike or fear a tumultuous existence. The school superintendent, the city hospital administrator, the director of a welfare agency, as well as the head of a state mental hospital, often finds himself today in the path of a hurricane, lashed by the winds of public demand for better service, the cries of groups with vested interests, and the indignation of taxpayers. But this is the price of public leadership: one has to give more, risk more, attempt more, face up to more. But there is, in compensation, the opportunity to accomplish more; in a sense, to live more intensely. One will certainly not be the spectator with a pale existence, but be right in the middle of the arena, matching wits with many an adversary. The stakes are high, and one can succeed mightily or fail mightily. One can affect—for good or ill—the lives of many, both public and staff, rather than just a few selected clients, patients, or students.

Success can be deeply gratifying for the top leader since he can affect an institution profoundly. He can be both the administrator and the affective leader. As administrator, he can actively shape policy at all levels. More than anyone else, he represents the hospital to the public and gives the institution its identity and form. As affective leader, he can help establish the climate of relationships between personnel and staff and between staff and patients. His successes may be measured along any one of these dimensions.

The path of the senior author to the superintendency of a state hospital may illustrate some of the attractions of such a position even for someone whose background was an academic one. As research director at Massachusetts Mental Health Center, he became deeply involved in the early 1950s in studying the effect of total hospital organization on patient care and treatment in several institutions that were shifting rapidly from custodial establishments to therapeutic communities.[8] In the course of these studies he noted that, generally, most psychiatrists devoted untold hours to learning how to change patients but very little time to learning how to change the institutions that house the ill. The so-called medical model with its emphasis on one-to-one relationships often narrowed their range, and they resisted recognizing the importance of environment in the genesis and the cure of their patients' difficulties. They were rarely if ever exposed in any detail to the concepts of milieu therapy during their in-hospital training. Their period of responsibility for a ward or program was all too brief, but considered sufficient for future needs. Unfortunately, this experience generally pertained to maintaining the social organization as it was, rather than changing it to something they might have wanted it to be. Changes of this sort were not expected to be the province of the clinician or the researcher, but of the senior administrator.

Thus, for a researcher who had long been interested in studying change in mental hospitals, the opportunity to implement his ideas in a difficult but vitally important sector of patient treatment—the state hospital—represented an irresistible challenge. Moreover, a research career in and of itself has closer links to the role of hospital superintendent than might be ordinarily expected. Success in research leads inevitably to administration in research. The more questions asked and vigorously pursued (and perhaps answered), the larger is the team of investigators; the more fiscal and personnel problems, the greater is the preoccupation with the details of organization—in other words, with administration.

Administration of the hospital itself can thus be a logical step in a career in which active pursuit of research has been the central mode. The hospital administrator is in truth in a most powerful position not only to aid the research interests of those in his organization, but also to appreciate problems in social psychiatry that escape others, to cultivate the creative resources of the many individuals around him, and to enhance the climate of inquisitiveness, of scholarship, and of resolution to find answers. Furthermore, he can so manage his organization, under reasonably favorable circumstances, that a considerable portion of his working time can be spent in truly creative work. Granted, he is no longer at the bench level, but he can have great satisfactions in personal involvement along a broad front of exciting innovations and investigations.

The administrator interested in research needs people, imaginative and dedicated people, to share his research and development approach to hospital improvement. Since few staff workers in large state institutions know this area well, he has a mammoth educational task before him. Basically, there are two ways in which an organization can obtain people with so-called principal investigator skills. One is to recruit trained workers from universities and laboratories; the other is to train them from the ground up. Both approaches were to be used at Boston State.

Many aspects of development at Boston State were congruent with the kind of overall orientation the senior author was to bring to the hospital. During his superintendency from 1945 to 1963,

Dr. Walter Barton had taken great strides toward transforming the formerly bleak custodial atmosphere of a large state institution to one with a more dynamic ambiance, including as he did the introduction of several community-oriented programs, such as home treatment,[9] day hospitals, and an outpatient clinic. The inpatient census had been significantly reduced from an overwhelming peak of three thousand to a more manageable twenty-four hundred with hope that much more could still be done. Over the years, the hospital had established a tradition of analytically oriented psychotherapy and making use of available educational resources, both of which gave it an academic orientation unusual for a state institution. Moreover, it had already carried out a number of important studies, thereby laying the foundation for a substantial and vigorous research program.

At the same time it became readily apparent that the new superintendent would face in this new job problems that were far greater than any he had ever encountered before. It was one thing to be involved with planning more treatment-oriented programs and stimulating research at a small, tightly knit university hospital. It was quite another to take over the leadership of a large, cumbersome institution, spread over many acres. The very physical dispersal represented an obstacle to integrated staff effort and a sense of cohesion. Many buildings were old and not easily rehabilitated, exacerbating the feeling of impoverishment so often found in state hospitals. Also, whatever its advantage in richness of staff when compared with other large mental hospitals, the manpower shortage was still tremendous.

And finally, to anticipate our story a bit, we soon realized that one of the greatest obstacles to be overcome was the ingrained attitude of staff itself, combined with the many external rigidities that meshed so neatly with bureaucratic personalities. A large hospital—either state, municipal, or private—is a ponderous system beset with tradition, laden with old ways of doing things, overburdened with chronic patients, flooded by tides of new admissions, shackled by rules, regulations, and legal restrictions, and suffering from a sense of inadequacy and deprivation.

Our emotional and intellectual reactions during the initial months at Boston State when confronted with the full impact of a large state organization soon synthesized to form one pervasive feeling: "Move, ye ponderous thing." Sometimes we experienced this challenge as an exhilarating opportunity, at other times, as a depressing, overwhelming task. Only slowly did we realize that we were encountering problems that were not unique to the hospital itself but in a large measure were part and parcel of the urban crisis of our times.

In the following text, we have tried to conceptualize our experiences in a way that would be most germane to persons interested in organizational change of any kind. Whatever success this book may achieve as a manual of instruction for present and future administrators matters considerably less than the possibility that it may encourage others with greater ability to contribute to the presently impoverished literature and to turn the attention of those interested in social and institutional change to the problems —and rewards—of leadership in human-service organizations.

The major themes around which this book is organized concern several sets of opposing polarities, each with its own valid claims for recognition by the administrator during the transitional period of reorganization. Some of these contrapositions include:

Centralization versus decentralization. Here we are concerned with the specific organizational challenge of breaking down a large, centrally administered organization into smaller, more comprehensive and autonomous subunits (see chapter 4). We are also concerned here, as we are throughout the text, with the even more difficult problem of suffusing involvement and initiative-taking at all levels of the organization. Issues in reconciling the needs for, and merits of, some forms of centralization are dealt with in terms of particular services and in terms of the role of top management in providing directional spark and thrust.

Unified philosophy versus multiple ideologies. Many organizations develop over time their own way of doing things, be it educating children, rehabilitating prisoners, or treating the sick. A substantial part of our narrative deals with the problems attendant to introducing a more pluralistic approach, not only in the direct treatment of patients but also in administrative practices in general. In this context, we were confronted with the larger polarities of intellectual dogmatism and organizational rigidity at one extreme and intellectual anarchy and administrative chaos at the other.

Equal distribution of resources versus special concentrations of wealth. In the economy of scarcity that afflicts our large public organizations, there is, understandably, tremendous momentum toward fair and equal distribution of staff and money commensurate with particular client burdens. At the same time, the development of an innovative service often needs intensive and unequal early cultivation in order to flourish. We deal with the organizational storms and stresses arising from these conflicting values in many sections of the text but particularly in the chapter on the development of an adolescent service.

Professional domain versus use of volunteers. No complaint is heard more frequently in our service organizations than "we have too few staff." Yet professionals are often loathe to welcome untrained but enthusiastic persons as collaborators in performing functions hitherto deemed, rightly or wrongly, the special province of highly trained persons. Here, our own strong bias for volunteer assistance is challenged by the intense and diverse arguments against the maximum use of lay citizens.

Underlying many of these and other polarities to be described is the larger one involving the *proper combination and juxtaposition of change and stability.* Both are badly needed in organizational life. If one moves too rapidly, even though the aims are worthy, much good can be swept aside in the path toward progress and staff can become so unsettled or disturbed that the move may prove to be dangerous or ineffective, or both. If one moves too slowly, staff may remain emotionally comfortable, but clients may suffer. It is intellectually much easier either to support the preservation of the status quo or to be in favor of immediate, total change. The harder task is to introduce less precipitous, but more lasting change, a process which above all entails helping staff and public develop their own capacities for growth.

Before turning to our first chapter, let us give a brief description of Boston State Hospital itself and its status in 1963, when this story began.

Boston State was established in 1839 as the first municipal mental institution in the United States. Since then it has served as the major public psychiatric facility for residents of Boston, and is located on the near fringes of that city. Large, rambling, spread over some two hundred and thirty acres of green and roadway, the hospital is visually a history of institutional architecture, ranging from a few wooden Victorian buildings to a new brick and glass "modern" edifice, so popular in the 1950s.

Since the hospital serves all of Boston, the patient population reflects the ethnic and racial diversity of that city. Although a majority of patients are lower-middle-class Catholic, of Irish and Italian descent, there is a substantial representation from the Protestant, black, and Jewish communities. Indeed, the immediate environment of the hospital was for many years a Jewish enclave, although recently black immigration and white emigration have radically altered the character of the community. Like so many cities, this area has been undergoing chaotic change with a rapid depletion of more affluent and stable groups, a sudden influx of multiproblem families, and a sharp rise in community tension.

In 1963, Boston State had a staff of twelve hundred and an inpatient population of some twenty-four hundred, consisting mainly of chronic patients in custodial or semicustodial status. That same year some twenty-five hundred admissions were processed, largely in one old building that held about one hundred and eighty beds. An outpatient clinic, three day units, and a home treatment facility helped serve the eight hundred thousand residents in Boston State's domain.

These brief statistics about the patients and staff hardly convey the flavor of the hospital. In a sense, Boston State was like an archeological find, with relics from different historic eras resting on each other. Thus, there were chronic patients who had lived in the hospital thirty years or more eating side by side with acute patients for whom the hospital represented not a lifelong home, but a few days' or weeks' interlude. Even more important, and relevant to our later analysis, were the differences among staff. Many of the staff, particularly among the attendants, supervising nurses, and various maintenance departments, had been employees for many years. They were deeply identified with keeping "law and order" and had little interest in the various training and research programs which they often viewed as obstacles to getting the work done. Working next to them were psychiatrists, nurses, psychologists, and social workers, who were interested in teaching and learning about psychiatric techniques. Many of these were younger people who would only be at the hospital for a short time to complete their training. Some of the seniors among them were drawn to Boston State by the magnet of Dr. Barton's vigorous efforts to improve the institution and had a particularly strong interest in the teaching of psychotherapy and psychodynamics. Added to this mix was the new layer of personnel to be attracted by our administration.

The reader will quickly see the similarities between the hospital and the urban city. In both instances, the innovative young must live side by side with the tradition-oriented old; the academic types with the doers; the transient with the permanent.

Each of these changes connected with many other facets of the internal organization and of the hospital's relations with the community. Let us turn now to some concepts and techniques of change itself in a large organizational structure.

REFERENCES

1. M. Jones, *The Therapeutic Community* (New York: Basic Books, 1963).

2. A. Stanton and M. Schwartz, *The Mental Hospital* (New York: Basic Books, 1954).

3. W. Caudill, *The Psychiatric Hospital as a Small Society* (Cambridge, Mass.: Harvard University Press, 1958).

4. H. A. Wilmer, "Toward a Definition of a Therapeutic Community," *American Journal of Psychiatry* 114(1958): 824–34.

5. L. Bellak, ed., *Handbook of Community Psychiatry and Community Mental Health* (New York: Grune and Stratton, 1964), especially "Comprehensive Community Psychiatry Program at City Hospital."

6. L. Linn, "Some Aspects of a Psychiatric Program in a Voluntary General Hospital," in ibid.

7. *The Executive Role Constellation* (Cambridge, Mass.: Division of Research, Harvard Business School, 1965).

8. M. Greenblatt, R. York, and E. L. Brown, eds. *From Custodial to Therapeutic Care in a Mental Hospital* (New York: Russell Sage Foundation, 1955).

9. L. Wiener, A. Becker, and T. T. Friedman, eds., *Home Treatment: Spearhead of Community Psychiatry* (Pittsburgh: University of Pittsburgh Press, 1967).

PART I

Concepts and Techniques of Change

CHAPTER 1

Within the Institution

The opportunity to effect institutional change is one of the great attractions and fascinations of the administrator's role. The good and sufficient compensation for the mass of details he must attend to is the satisfaction of altering the organization in a favorable direction. But what are the techniques of effecting change? How well do they work? What are the expected stresses on the individual and on the system, and how do we handle their consequences? Or, to be more specific, where do we start? How fast shall we go? How many fronts should be activated at the same time? What are the major resistances? And, how much change can the system absorb without excessive creaks and groans?

Stimulating Organizational Creativity

Where progressive institutional change is desired, the central variable is the administrator's attitude toward organizational creativity. Since change can be made only by individuals, he must question how much creativity already exists among the people in the organization, how it can be elicited, and how much effort he is willing to exert.

Our first assumption at Boston State was that the potential for creativity was vast, but that it was locked up by innumerable individual and organizational barriers. With roughly twelve hundred people on the staff, it seemed that a very small additional effort by all of them could solve a great many problems. How much more effort would people be willing to give if their interest were stimulated, if their wish to create were activated, and if they found new, deeply satisfying channels of expression?

This assumption was fortified by our repeated observation of how individuals poorly placed within a system or poorly managed would fail to deliver. However, when the same people were reassigned to jobs more suitable to their inner needs, and were shown appreciation and given rewards, they would often perform remarkably well. Further, time and again we observed that institutions as a whole can rise to dramatic heights of efficiency and productivity when proper inspiration is provided. To provide the inspiration is the function of "the man in charge," as well as to motivate, to encourage, to stretch the potential, to help make staff happy and productive, doing the job it does best and not necessarily the one assigned by bureaucratic rigidity.

A task, then, of primary importance at Boston State would be to make a diagnosis of every individual and group in the system, asking first what was holding them back, how to unlock the door to the energy storehouses within, and how to stimulate creativity in a large staff working under difficult conditions.

Where to start? We believed we should deal initially with those people and problems that came to us first in the natural functioning of the system, attempting to build individual relationships with the persons immediately around us. However, it was also imperative to look even deeper, to scrutinize and study the more complex and subtle interrelationships and functions of the organization. In doing so, we soon became aware that only a small portion of the submerged potential of the organization could be freed by our own direct efforts, but that a chain reaction could be set up by stimulating a variety of people in key formal and informal positions. They, in turn, could elicit creativity in their orbit, and so on, successively throughout the institution. One World Health Organization technical report[1] stresses a similar kind of thinking in describing the therapeutic atmosphere of a treatment system:

The most important single factor in the efficacy of the treatment given in a mental hospital appears to the committee to be an intangible element which can only be described as its atmosphere. . . . As in the community at large, one of the characteristic aspects of the psychiatric hospital is the type of relationship between people that are to be found within it. The nature of the relationship between the medical director and his staff will be reflected between the psychiatric staff and the nurses, and finally in the relationship not only between the nurses and the patients, but between the patients themselves.

The Pace of Change

The pace of change, as well as the focus of change is, to a large extent, left to the judgment of the administrator. Should he go fast, or should he go slow? Whatever the decision, it should be made with dispatch, because it is one of the first issues on which a new administrator must take a position.

The advantages of swift change are manifold. First, it demonstrates as early as possible that the new administration means business. Second, it develops an atmosphere of action and movement. Third, it accustoms staff as early as possible to rapid change as a philosophical principle of management. In the case of Boston State, there was still another advantage. It gave outside observers the impression that the hospital was a place where vital things were happening, that it was worth watching because it was in motion. To those interested in social change, nothing is so fascinating as a large organization on the move, especially if it is a treatment organization. We felt that if our changes were rapid and progressive, we could stimulate the interest of people sufficiently for them to come nearer to take a closer look. And the closer look was often the first step in the recruitment of new, high-quality staff.

Despite an administrator's decision to move quickly, there still exist many factors that continually slow his progress. The many intrapsychic reasons for resistance have been well documented in the literature on psychodynamics and need not be pursued in any depth here. For most people, change is upsetting and anxiety-provoking, especially if their future roles are not clearly visualized. Old reliable methods of doing things carry great security, and neither an individual nor a whole system that is comfortable is quick to welcome change that may be threatening.

The amount of anxiety that is engendered by change can be enormous. Some people become sick. Absenteeism goes way up. Some threaten to quit; others do quit. Some unleash hostility against their superiors and associates. Predictions of disaster or doom are rampant. Outside agents and agencies, such as family, public officials, or influential lay citizens, are called in by those who are threatened to help return the system to its former stability. Even the press may be contacted to announce "the terrible things that are going on," and the administrator may face physical danger or see his good name threatened.

Generally, most of the resistance against change bears little relationship to the soundness of the change advocated, but relates instead to the types of anxieties that change as such produces. Change, therefore, has to be coupled with a program of anxiety reduction. This is a kind of administrative therapy for individuals and groups. Participation in numerous planning sessions and consultations aimed at working through these tensions, the delegation of responsibility to a large number of people, a system of appeals for aggrieved individuals, clarification of steps in initiating change —these are a few of the techniques available.

Anxiety cannot be reduced to zero. Indeed, a certain amount of tension is necessary for continued productivity. Furthermore, in many instances there is a subtle attempt at seduction by some staff to involve administration in what amounts to their psychotherapy. The personality problems of such people are deeper than situational. In giving a kind of administrative therapy to a person in trouble, there is a point beyond which it is wise not to go, or the whole process of change becomes bogged down in the endless psychological needs of problematic individuals. What must not be overlooked is the fact that change, and rapid change especially, will hurt some people no matter how well planned. There *is* a price to pay. Moreover, those individuals who need too much help and attention in order to negotiate change are probably better off in an organization that is not in sharp transition.

What are the costs of going slow? Against the advantage of minimal disruption and disturbance of staff the slow pace of change has great disadvantage in that great efforts have to be expended to educate staff to the *need* and motivate them to a *desire* for change. In a rigid, entrenched system, both initiative and resistance by staff may depend basically on their wishes for comfort and their belief that if they resist long enough, this wild innovator also will go away, like a long line before him. And while waiting for the staff to come around—and the wait can be very long—the administrator is getting little done. In this day and age of extraordinarily great lag in proper treatment for the mentally ill, we simply cannot afford to trade the patient's health for staff convenience. If, indeed, one wishes to provide optimum care as quickly as possible to as many patients as possible, then one must train staff to a sense of urgency, to rapid achievement.

As a final point, the drive in the organization for change will depend, eventually, on the type of relationships that develop between the administrator and his staff. Relationships leading to trust and respect are forged by a long process of working together to overcome obstacles. In developing and shaping a working management team, going fast is more satisfactory than going slow, for if change is rapid, the relationships are charged or energized by the effort to adapt to moving events. The strengths and the weaknesses of the individuals in the group assert themselves immediately. The testing, the accommodations, and the internal rearrangement that are needed to make a hard-hitting and secure team take place much more rapidly. Those who cannot make the grade know it sooner rather than later and can step aside. For those who remain, the reward is great, for there is nothing like having worked and triumphed together through hard times.

How Many Fronts to Activate?

In the large mental hospital, treatment, training, and research exist on many fronts. Should one area be activated at a time, or as many as possible? The conservative approach is to take it one at a time, to do it well, to observe, to study, to draw conclusions for future reference. The more radical approach, however, is to activate many fronts at once. Here one sacrifices the careful nurturing necessary to push a given program through to success, to gamble that once a program is started individuals with true leadership capacity will seize the opportunity to emerge and take it over. When this happens, a good administrator will work primarily as a catalyst, with only an occasional attempt at "quality control." Once indigenous leadership is found, the detailed follow-through is left to others. This latter technique also capitalizes on the probability that one program will enhance another, especially true if a sense of excitement, challenge, or competition begins to take hold.

Our policy at Boston State was to activate many programs simultaneously. This led to many complaints: the new programs are draining staff time; they are exhausting resources; they are conflicting with each other, and so forth. We found we needed to spend much time with staff to explain that a system with many innovations under one roof was not only feasible, but was also obligatory for a hospital to grow in an integrated fashion.

One of the most difficult tasks was to persuade staff to take a long- rather than a short-term view of the allocation of personnel. It was understandably very hard for an already overburdened ward staff to accept the temporary loss of a nurse or aide so that she could participate in the development of a new program. The new program would put us in a better position to obtain research or demonstration funds, which, in turn, might eventually provide five or six additional people to help harrassed ward staff with their service tasks. This is precisely what could and did happen in many instances where a small service gamble properly directed into an area of rich research potential yielded significant patient benefits and a vigorous research and training program. (A description of how this works will be seen in the chapter on the adolescent service.)

Change and the Question of Structure

We have emphasized that the fostering of change was to be a cardinal value and that rapid change was to be implemented on many fronts. One kind of administrative style to foster change in a large organization is to use the bureaucratic structure that already exists and, where necessary, to add new lines of authority for new programs. Another style is to try to loosen up the rigid, hierarchical lines and to develop more flexible roles and ways of functioning among personnel.

We have already suggested that the first alternative would not have been syntonic with our goals. The very notion of a bureaucratic, tight organization contributes, especially as it functions undisturbed over time, to routine ways of doing things. In such a system, when staff are confronted with a problem, they decide to handle it on the basis of what was done in the past. Precedent is all-powerful; innovation is suspect. Even if one replaces the old, formal structure with a new one—and such a replacement is in practice extraordinarily difficult to achieve and devastating to staff morale—the old rigidities are likely to appear in new form within a very short time.

Faced with the problem of deciding on organizational form, we took the position of deemphasizing structure as such. Understandably, such an approach arouses great anxiety among staff. Hospital personnel are usually accustomed to working with a clear chain of command, where formal orders flow downward and buck-passing flows upward. The usual anxieties attendant to the deemphasis of structure were compounded at Boston State when staff learned that the new superintendent planned to bring in many new people within a relatively short time. One of the first staff reactions was that they needed structure to define the relationships between the new people and the old, and, in the case of programs, to define roles. It was astonishing how uncomfortable staff at *all* levels felt unless everything was defined by higher authority.

Such longing for the boss's decision often reflects considerable anxiety about the degree of support one will get from his superiors if one takes responsibility and, in doing so, makes mistakes. It is therefore important that a new director, especially in the initial phase of his administration, demonstrate in action that when trouble arises he will discourage the stultifying game of seeking authoritative mandate for every little move or act.

During the process of change at Boston State, the attitudes of staff frequently swung from a desire for strict authoritarian order on the one hand to the rejection of any order on the other. Complaints from the same person would alternate between "I want to know whom I take orders from" and "Why do I have to take orders from *him?*" The more ambivalence, the more such questions; but the very questioning of authority seemed to be an advance over former, blanket acquiescence.

In the course of time, we found that most staff could get used to a minimum, flexible kind of structure when they saw the advantage of this system. With such a system, we could implement new, worthwhile ideas more quickly and give more responsibility and reward to those who were willing to take initiative. There were, however, some staff who, by temperament, could not accept deemphasis of formal structure. They were often the same people who found the expectation of rapid change too anxiety-provoking. Again, many of these people needed considerable doses of "administrative therapy" to help them cope with the problems of transition.

Thus, deemphasis of structure amounted to deemphasis of hierarchy and control, reaffirmation of the flexibility of the system, and, finally, acceptance of the possibility of being secure and happy in a changing environment.

Open Communication

Hospitals that have a rigid chain of command usually have highly segregated networks of communication. Nurses speak only to nurses; doctors speak only to doctors, and so on. An institution committed to change must also be committed to free interdepartmental exchange. Indeed, there is empirical evidence that institutions receptive to innovation also have a high level of communication between departments.

Since the energy and direction of change derive initially from the top, the administrator interested in change must be particularly concerned about keeping *his* channels of communication open to all major arenas of the hospital. If communications from the administrator to personnel or from personnel to him are stopped by rigid departmental barriers, many staff members, especially low- or middle-level personnel, will never get a clear idea of the administrator's intentions. Nor will he get a clear picture of staff's feelings and reactions. If an open system does not operate, a solid relationship can never be developed between administration and staff.

Fortunately, with the deemphasis of structure at Boston State and the shift toward informality, it became possible to open up channels of communication to accomplish highly significant changes in attitudes. A case in point was the weekly meeting of the senior psychiatric group, which was being run almost like a session in group psychotherapy. For some years it had been implicit that the superintendent was not to be part of that group, even though much that transpired was of great import for hospital morale, policy formulation, and clinical-administrative cooperation. When the superintendent suggested that he would like to attend the meetings, he was told that he would have to wait for the group to clear him for admission. The senior psychiatrists were operating under the assumption that closed communication was desirable and that top clinical staff should properly meet by themselves. If they had any complaint or action they deemed relevant to administration, it would be reported to the superintendent by their appropriate leaders at an appropriate time. This way of doing business obviously prevented the superintendent from injecting his own ideas and feelings into the discussion process and tended to divide the hospital into two camps—one clinical and one administrative.

It did not take long to realize that this insistence on closed communication reflected friction between clinical staff and administration. It was our conviction that closed or highly formal procedures of communication would only exacerbate this negative feeling and that one way to resolve it would be to open the meeting wide, to talk together so we could more easily work together. When this belief was made known to staff, they reluctantly permitted the superintendent to attend as an observer; later, he was included as a participant. In the course of some two years, the meetings progressed by stages through covert and overt antagonism toward administration to a much greater degree of cooperation and good will. During the same period, the tenor of the meetings shifted from mainly expressions of dissatisfaction and complaint with minimal or no interest in corrective action, to emphasis on responsible action and problem-solving, with affective expression linked to a positive program. Eventually, with the shift of emphasis toward problem-solving, the new superintendent was voted moderator of the group.

First as participant and later as moderator, the superintendent's technique was to encourage the assumption of initiative, responsibility, and freedom to experiment with new ways of doing things: "Don't wait for orders, but try out your plan if those involved can agree to its merits, and, even if some think it may not have merit, it may still be worth trying." Because success had often been reached despite dire warnings, the administrator often displayed impatience with those who made gloomy predictions of disaster. Courage and boldness were praised, and it was openly assumed that those who tried out new ideas would certainly make some mistakes. Such mistakes not only were to be expected but were also even welcomed, since they would often add to knowledge and experience.

One important lesson learned was that opening communication often lessens the polarities between individuals and departments and reveals that members of a particular group are not necessarily all of one mind about controversial matters. Prior to attending the meetings, we frequently got reports that the senior staff felt thus-and-so about a particular idea, as though they all shared one opinion. After participating, we realized that there were considerable differences of opinion among them, with many who were assumed to oppose a new program actually in favor of it. In closed meetings, differences are often concealed either because people disagreeing with the "main line" are afraid to speak out, or because those differences that do occur are screened out by biased reporters.

Another lesson learned from the seniors' meetings was the importance of problem-solving as the logical end result of discussion and argument. In an overcrowded, understaffed, overworked, generally overwhelmingly large hospital, the crush of problems is so great that morale sags and the task seems hopeless. Group and individual complaining takes the place of corrective action, and problems pile up. Under such conditions, it is the job of the administrator to point the way toward continued action based on the conviction that most problems *can* be solved.

Problem-solving is an especially needed antidote in a hospital that concentrates on psychodynamics. Psychotherapeutically oriented staff members working with relatively intractable psychotic patients are accustomed, often with good reason, to concentrate on the why and wherefore of a patient's condition, even if a clear treatment plan cannot be designed. The same way of thinking can be easily transferred to institutional problems. One can spend endless time diagnosing why the problems exist and, unless prodded, never get on with finding a solution.

The End Run

Another technique used to loosen the formal organization was to permit the so-called end run, that is, the bypassing of one's immediate superior to deal directly with someone at a higher level. Let us first state the organizational problem for which the end run provides one partial solution.

When a new administrator of a large organization takes over, he is usually given a structure with inherited department heads and subheads, many of whom do not favor either his desire for change or his methods of achieving it. He must decide how much to recognize their authority in all matters pertaining to subordinates or how much to permit direct communication between lower-level staff and his office. It is a double-edged sword. On the one hand, if he allows all communication to be screened first through the department head, it may be difficult to know what is going on below that executive's level. On the other hand, if he permits subordinates to communicate directly with him, the effect on the department head may be devastating. This is especially true when a top lieutenant has had the full confidence and trust of the previous administrator. However, if the new director invariably blocks the end run and deals only with top lieutenants, it does not necessarily mean that, in return for such respect, they will interpret his philosophy properly, especially his concepts of innovation, creativity, and looser lines of administration, which many find so difficult to understand.

A new administrator who does not come from the ranks of the institution he now heads feels a need to learn early what is going on at lower levels and to learn this as quickly as possible. It was thus decided to permit selected end runs, despite their difficulties. It seemed wise to allow a certain degree of access to the front office directly, rather than always through formal channels or the procedure of grievance hearings. We anticipated that as confidence grew between the department heads and the new superintendent, tensions would be eased and the technique of the end run would be less needed. When end runs did occur, the department heads would not see them as an affront, but as a means of quick information transmittal with a minimum of red tape.

It must be pointed out, however, that the technique of the end run constitutes an inherent stress and if used unwisely can lead to two major abuses: (1) subordinates believe that the authority of the department head has been abrogated and so treat him with less respect, and (2) the department head fails to report to the director, or in various ways tries to turn over the reins of management to him. But despite these dangers, we believe the judicious acceptance of the end run is worth the gamble to the new administrator: not only will it keep him in touch with staff at all levels, but it will also keep *them* in touch with *him*. This is particularly important during the initial period of turmoil and disagreement that frequently occurs with change in top command.

Progressive Expectations

Without aims or challenges, an organization—and a hospital organization in particular—tends to slow down, and in fact, to run downhill. A technique to prevent what could be a relentless course of deterioration is to set up a progressive series of challenges to mobilize strength, to raise morale, and to produce cohesiveness.

These challenges may be hospital-wide, such as gearing up for accreditation or planning programs for decentralization into units, reduction of census, ward therapy, and reassignment of personnel to community tasks. Or the programs may apply to one ward, pavilion, or service, such as ward renovation, night hospitalization, and so on. In either case, the administrator should have in mind a series of progressive goals and accomplishments that can move the organization in the direction he has planned.

The series of goals need not have originated with the administrator. They can come from many sources and arise in many ways—through suggestions by staff, through recommendations by patients, or through application of knowledge of successful programs at other institutions. Or they can be the result of guidelines and orders handed down from the Department of Mental Health or through legislative action. It is very useful for the administrator to stress the outside source of ideas, particularly when they coincide with or strengthen internal directions. This can help to overcome staff's feeling that a given new program is merely the caprice of a single individual. Staff learn that the suggested innovations reflect a general movement that transcends the hospital, and that their implementation is essential if the institution wishes to maintain and improve its level of support from state or federal government. However, the administrator should not give grudging acquiescence to a program just because outsiders demand it. Such an attitude may help to consolidate feeling between staff and their leader against a common, external force, but it will reduce severely the enthusiasm and creativity attendant to program implementation.

Whatever the sources of new ideas, their development requires considerable discussion and argument, so that many points of view can be aired and decisions shared as to the appointment of planning committees to initiate activity. Such discussion helps convince staff that they, too, may share the philosophy of progressive expectations. It also allows them to participate in the details and timing of implementation. Finally, in trying to arrive at consensus, discussion often turns negativism into positive action. There is often a point when staff feel that the problem has been talked to death and that they might as well get on with action. Fulfilling the expectation of progressive change becomes less painful than further arguments.

When, however, staff show so much resistance that one cannot count on them to meet the new expectation, the setting of a second expectation may accelerate the acceptance of the first. Sometimes the second expectation is so controversial that it dwarfs the first in the degree of opposition and resistance it arouses. Staff's energy goes into opposing the second idea, and they thus become more amenable to the first. Compared with the new challenge, the earlier expectation may seem a good deal more moderate than when it stood alone.

If progressive expectations are well arranged, it may happen that fulfillment of the second expectation demands the simultaneous implementation of the first. To illustrate: in 1963, Boston State was largely segregated as to sex. On arrival, the superintendent announced a goal of integration of men and women within the limitations of ward and building architecture. In some buildings housing only women, it was feasible to have men on one floor and women on another. In other buildings, ward layout permitted women on one side and men on another, often with a common day room between. In still other buildings, it was possible to have men and women on the same ward in different rooms, with one or more patients of the same sex per room.

The goal of integration was met lackadaisically and only here and there. In most areas, it was blocked by resistance based either on "inadequate bathroom facilities," fear that in exchanging patients with other services one would get the bad end of the deal, preference by ward chiefs for treating one or the other sex, lack of conviction that integration was better for patients than segregation, or sheer inertia.

When it became apparent that integration would not proceed much further on its own, we evoked another hospital goal—decentralization. Decentralization—or unitization as it is often called —meant admitting patients of both sexes from a given geographic area to a given hospital service and treating them on the same service throughout their career as patients. By its very nature, the second goal presupposed implementation of the first goal— integration of men and women—as a precondition to its full accomplishment.

Infusion of Ideas from Without

Most professional organizations depend on intellectual stimulation for growth and to make them receptive to change. Mental hospitals, particularly, have a tendency to become parochial in their attitudes unless there is active input from outside the system. Despite their need to think in broader terms, particularly in this era of new approaches to treatment, some staff still have little interest in the world around them, in the ideas of professionals in other parts of the country. It seems extraordinarily difficult for them to leave their offices and their families, take a plane, or even visit other institutions just a few miles away. Yet, in our experience, it is rare for a professional to visit another establishment without gaining important new perspectives on what was being done at home, or acquiring altogether new ideas of what is both feasible and advantageous to try.

Such visiting should not be limited to one or even a few top-level professionals. Apart from the drain on their time from frequent traveling, the hospital's public image may become too narrowly identified with a few personalities. Most important, top echelon tends to talk only with top echelon, with the risk that a less-than-full picture of what is really going on in the other institutions is obtained. A group of young colleagues encouraged by the administrator to travel to other facilities can broaden the hospital's image, bring back many new ideas, and ultimately make the institution richer and more varied.

For example, when decentralization was being considered, three of our younger psychiatrists visited facilities that had already unitized—Clarinda State Hospital in Iowa,[2] Fort Logan in Colorado,[3] and Kansas State Hospital.[4] As a result of their trip, they obtained such a positive view of the advantages of unitization that they were able to impart their enthusiasm to the rest of staff at a hospital-wide meeting and thus hastened the step toward formulating plans for decentralization. In like manner, a visit to Ypsilanti State Hospital in Michigan highlighted the value of work therapy for geriatric patients and encouraged efforts toward establishing sheltered workshops.

Greater Participation and the Delegation of Decision-making

Although we have emphasized that the top administrator must provide the central energy and direction for change, the subtlety of his art lies in doing it at the very time he is encouraging others to join him in initiating change. The issue here is more specific than simply encouraging creativity and initiative at various levels. It concerns the administrator's technique in involving others in planning and developing new programs. In doing this, he must steer a narrow course. If he takes too much decision-making upon himself, he risks the danger of being regarded as a heavy-handed autocrat and evokes the hostility and resistance that often accompany the response to such authority. If, however, the decision-making process becomes too diffuse, the central thrust can be weakened and the feeling of movement slowed down by a morass of crosscutting wishes and interests.

The first danger faces the superintendent of a mental hospital more poignantly than it does the administrator of a general hospital. In most state hospitals, the superintendent has czarlike powers; all responsibility and authority formally belong to him. In general hospitals, the top executive supervises mainly administrative areas, while the responsibility for large clinical domains is vested in powerful chiefs of staff in surgery, medicine, and so on. Theoretically, the state hospital superintendent could make every major decision himself; indeed, if he wished he could approve every letter sent out of the hospital or every memorandum distributed within it. Practically, however, this is not feasible and certainly not desirable. Were the administrator to follow such an obsessive path, he would soon find that the substance of his ideas would be lost in their execution, since change cannot be successfully implemented by staff members who feel controlled and mistrusted.

Yet the second danger is equally real. If he follows the model of the general hospital administrator and delegates too much power to the clinical director, nursing director, and so on, he may find that he has attenuated his own ability to influence the system. This is particularly the case when an administrator has inherited many of his top lieutenants. He is then faced with the difficult task of initiating movement while simultaneously trying to win over their trust and enthusiasm in planning and implementing change.

How does he accomplish this? The resident-training program at Boston State Hospital is a case in point. One of our first decisions in attempting to reorganize this all-important activity was to establish a committee—the psychiatric executive committee—consisting initially of two clinical directors, the assistant superintendent, and the superintendent. The clear implications of this move were that decisions about the training program would not be made solely by the superintendent. Nor, as was formerly the case, would they be delegated solely to the clinical directors. Although there were very good reasons for expanding this important committee beyond these four members, the clinical directors were so accustomed to controlling the domain, they would have interpreted the addition of eight more members as an autocratic act aimed at reducing their own powers.

Such an expansion did eventually occur. It required gentle assistance, accompanied by repeated discussions of the pros and cons of each new addition, modulated and timed in such a manner that it could be tolerated and accepted within the bounds of a growing relationship of confidence and respect.

The expansion did not represent simply a "court-packing" operation for the sake of bringing into the decision process those with ideas similar to our own, although there were elements of this. Primarily, the new members represented sources of new ideas and stimulation. We were gradually moving away from debates about power or conflicts between sharply polarized ideologies toward a much freer exchange and broader participation in decision-making.

Bench Strength

No matter how great the new director's efforts are to win the loyalty and affection of his staff, there still remain some who cannot accept rapid change, or whose temperamental or ideological differences with administration are so great that no working resolution is possible. In such cases it may be necessary to replace these lieutenants. To do so with as little disruption to the organization as possible, the administrator must have "bench strength."

The term *bench,* borrowed from sports, refers to the number of trained persons in an organization capable of filling positions that occur in the natural process of evolution. If the administrator lacks bench strength, he is virtually at the mercy of his personnel. If his bench is strong, he has many favorable options open to him. He is not compelled to work endlessly with recalcitrant people, and he does not have to be unreasonably cautious about upsetting a staff member for fear he might leave. He can operate with a sense of inner freedom and choice. When the bench is strong, staff know that his interest in them does not reflect desperation. If they falter or resign, they can be replaced; they will leave no permanent serious vacuum. They get the message, and they are on their mettle to deliver.

The techniques of developing bench strength are complex. In order to know who is potential leadership material, the administrator must have wide contacts throughout the ranks of personnel, with opportunities to cultivate personally those with unusual talent. This highlights the advantages of open communication, as well as the disadvantages of a rigid chain of command.

The development of bench strength also requires that every sensitive position be made as attractive as possible. As an illustration, some hospitals cannot fill the position of assistant superintendent because this post is often routine and uninspiring. It may be necessary to cut sharply the monotonous duties of this job, to give the incumbent generous allotments of time to study and create, and to provide him, in addition, with stimulating supervision. In this way the second-in-command will begin to grow and his improved morale will yield tenfold benefits to the hospital. Because of his increased worth, he will be sought after by other institutions, but many other people will now clamor for the job should he decide to leave.

Bench strength may further be developed by recruiting people from without. The wider the administrator's personal contacts outside the organization, the more likely he is to know people with the requisite potential who might be interested in playing on his team. It pays in long-term recruiting dividends if the administrator keeps up his outside contacts by way of letters, telephone calls, or visits with colleagues en route to professional meetings. Since these activities often do not pay any immediate dividends, it might seem to casual observers that they are unrelated to the administrator's "real work." Yet, such contacts are crucially related to the building of the kind of team that can implement his growing program. And like all good construction, this development requires time, patience, and the steadfast adherence to a master plan.

REFERENCES

1. *Expert Committee on Mental Health, Third Report,* World Health Organization, Technical Report Series no. 73 (Geneva, 1953), pp. 17–18.

2. L. B. Garcia, "The Clarinda Plan: An Ecological Approach to Hospital Organization," *Mental Hospitals* 11 (1960): 30–31.

3. E. Bonn and A. Kraft, "The Fort Logan Mental Health Center: Genesis and Development," *Journal of Fort Logan Mental Health Center* 1 (1963): 17–27.

4. G. W. Jackson and F. V. Smith, "A Proposal for Mental Hospital Reorganization: The Kansas Plan," *Mental Hospitals* 12 (1961): 5–8.

CHAPTER 2

The Institution and the Community

No matter what internal changes are planned for an organization, they can be either weakened or enhanced depending on the institution's relations with the community. For example, training programs for personnel can be enlarged and improved if positive relations have been established with institutions of higher learning. In like manner, plans that involve the immediate community can be strengthened by gaining their endorsement prior to initiating the project. In short, favorable change in an institution is dependent on a fusion of two worlds—the one within and the one without.

In the past, the typical state hospital, like many large, public-service organizations, tried to maintain as sharp a boundary with the community as possible. The hospital made little attempt to enlighten the community about its operation or to find out how the community could help it with its tasks. Funding came largely from only one source—the state government—and no effort was made to raise money elsewhere. Nor did the hospital cultivate collaboration with academic centers, even though, in many instances, such intellectual stimulation was available if sought.

We need not detail any further the emotional, financial, and intellectual insularity of the large custodial hospital since it has been described vividly by Goffman[1] and others.[2] Fortunately, Boston State had, for almost twenty years, been moving away from such isolation. To continue and sometimes to accelerate this movement, we took the steps described below.

Living Out

One manifestation of staff retreat from the community is their tendency to live on the hospital grounds. It is as though they too have need for withdrawal, an attitude similar to that of the patients they serve. For live-in staff, life within the hospital has very special benefits. They avoid the hustle and bustle of the world outside. They can meet their living needs with minimum effort, with few of the problems of running a household. Rent and meals are cheap. Laundry is done without cost on the hospital grounds, and there are no monthly bills for utilities. Living quarters usually come completely furnished, and even such vital necessities as drugs and medical care are free. It is a simplified existence, unfettered by the many worries and routines of everyday life.

Living-in facilities are often provided by administration on the basis that they make it easier to recruit personnel and, what is more important, to keep them. In living together, staff become part of a private club with strong group spirit, sharing around-the-clock goals, gossip, and excitement of hospital life.

Undoubtedly, this arrangement does have real advantages in terms of staff morale. But it also has grave disadvantages. For one, it forces the administrator into the role of landlord, with all its cares and hazards—problems of maintenance, disputes among staff for favored dwellings, and the like. These issues come to the administrator for resolution when his time would be better occupied with the affairs of patient care. From staff's point of view, their problems in dealing with the administrator as their "boss" are now compounded by having to deal with the same person as landlord.

The main disadvantage, however, of staff living on the grounds is that it diminishes their contact with the community. If they live out, they can learn how the community feels about the hospital and are in a much better position to interpret the hospital to the community. Moreover, they need that distance to take a critical look at the hospital, to be less blind to its shortcomings. "The last person to discover the nature of water is the fish."

Although Boston State did not have a large live-in staff population, there were still enough to make the philosophy of living out a controversial issue. The first step the administrator took was to exemplify this philosophy by practice: he did not move into the superintendent's house, but continued to live in his own home, several miles away from the hospital. Furthermore, he announced that the superintendent's residence was to be converted to a transitional facility for patients from the hospital to the community, thereby helping to break down the barrier between the two worlds.

The decision to live off the grounds set the precedent for some staff to move out, even though the administrator did not actively press them to do so. Not only did this liberate them from the insularity of hospital life, but it also freed space—without disrupting patients—to bring more of the outside world into the hospital, especially in the form of independently financed research projects and university-affiliated programs.

Thus, several floors of one attractive building were vacated and the space converted into offices for research personnel. Eventually, living quarters in three other buildings were emptied, thereby releasing even more room to establish working areas for personnel connected with new programs.

The foregoing illustrates how a circle of segregation can be converted into a spiral of integration. If staff members live in, they tend to be isolated from the world outside, which inhibits them from obtaining the intellectual and emotional stimulation they need for growth. If staff members live out, their involvement in the outside world grows and provides room for that world to move in. This, in turn, brings new resources to help the patient move into the community and to attract further outside interest in the hospital, thus enriching the lives of those who are already there.

Money and the Community

However generous the state may be, most public-service institutions, and especially large mental hospitals, are always in need of funds. Not only are allocations by most state legislatures on a low level, but they are also rigidly circumscribed by administrative rules and regulations. The line budget of a state system makes transfers between categories extremely difficult, if not impossible. For example, if X amount of money has been allotted for supplies, a portion of it cannot be used for salaries, or vice versa. Requests for new funds require new justifications, and approval is often so long in coming that worthwhile projects tend to die of neglect. Salary schedules are so inflexible that no leeway is provided to add extra incentives for recruiting staff of unusual caliber. Purchasing restrictions require awards to lowest bidders, often resulting in merchandise of shoddy quality, with subsequent large repair and maintenance costs. Delays in payment of salaries because of red tape complicate life further.

Many of the state rules have a rational basis in that they are aimed to curb corruption and waste. However, they often serve to reinforce the bureaucratic rigidity in a state system, not least because they can readily be used as a convenient excuse for those staff who dislike a new idea. It requires some persistence and skill on the part of the new administrator to disentangle the objective ruling from a staff member's interpretation of it, or from his distortion of someone else's interpretation "down at the central department." One of the administrator's most frustrating initial experiences is the constant refrain, "You can't change this, the state won't allow it."

But what can be done?

With regard to the low level of appropriations, history has shown that state funds can be increased. Educational campaigns by professional nonprofit associations and interested lay groups can mobilize a spirited public which, in turn, can forcibly bring these issues to the attention of legislators. The administrator can participate in such movements in a variety of ways. This does not mean that he, or the institution, has to become immersed in politics. It does mean, however, that the institution can, and often should, undertake programs of information for legislators. Lectures, pamphlets, or regular tours of inspection of the facility can help them in arriving at informed judgments. In our experience, conscientious legislators not only need and want the information, but they are also grateful for it.

In some instances, the cultivation of a local state senator or representative may lead to his introducing and backing legislative implementation for desired projects. However, the institution need not limit itself to seeking new resources from the state government. Relatively great additions to the budget can be made by working with other agencies—federal funding groups, private foundations, business organizations, and citizens' groups, to name a few.

The question may be posed that even if money can be raised in this way, should it be? Should a public institution seek funds from diverse sources, or should it take the position that it gets money only from the state? Our contention is that the state cannot possibly provide all that is necessary to treat patients or clients properly, that financing must be multiple, and that energetic pursuit of funds is the hospital's business. Moreover, outside funds are likely to increase flexibility in the range of spending, thus ameliorating one of the most noxious problems in fiscal management.

Who does the fund-raising?

It is fundamentally impossible for the administrator alone to cultivate all the resources, to do all the planning, and to carry out all the work attendant to pursuing this goal. It is necessary, therefore, in this instance as it is in others, to broaden the base of participation by delegating some of this responsibility to staff. Not only will this result in a far greater return for the institution, but it will also constitute a formidable training experience. There is nothing so useful in teaching staff the value of a dollar, or the problems of fiscal responsibility, as involving them in the art of raising money. Furthermore, such participation is an excellent cure for chronic complaints about the lack of money.

At the outset of the new administration, staff learned that fund-raising is everybody's business and that fund-raising from a variety of sources is especially relevant to developing programs in community psychiatry. Although the state will, and does, finance some of these programs, its constant financial burden just to maintain more traditional inpatient and outpatient services is tremendous. More flexible and less burdened financial sources are often better able and more willing to underwrite programs in this relatively new field. With the shared responsibility of raising money for *their* hospital, staff will soon learn the art of coordinating ideas with funding agencies. For example, an innovative program that offers an alternative to hospitalization is likely to interest the federal government; an enterprising idea in halfway houses or summer camps can capture the imagination of private citizens, and so forth.

Finally, something should be said about raising money from staff. Generosity of employees in occasionally dipping into their pockets to provide something for their impoverished patients is well known. In our experience, this is found more in the ranks of attendants and nurses with low salaries than among higher-paid personnel. Some staff, however, fear that any relief to the state through their donations might decrease state appropriations, and so withhold their individual contributions. Yet, granted that such revenue from staff is small, it is nevertheless important to cultivate the spirit of giving if they are to participate enthusiastically in the effort to raise funds from outside sources.

Interrelationships with the Community

All institutions, and especially state mental hospitals, have a tendency to wall themselves off from other groups, to think about the world within the organization as *us* and the world outside as *them*. It may be necessary for *us* to have formal relations with *them* on this or that matter of joint concern, but the truly close feelings are reserved for *us*. These difficulties between *us* and *them* are usually magnified when the hospital deals with the immediate community. Outsiders who wish to visit the hospital, or to participate in a treatment activity on a volunteer basis, or to finance a new project are often viewed with suspicion. "What are their motives?" "Will they upset the patients?" "Will they want to control the program they're giving money for?"

The idea of staff going out into the community often meets with as much opposition as the idea of the community coming into the hospital. It is amazing how quickly something outside institutional limits can be identified as "body alien" or something that is "not our business." To certain staff their business is seen only as taking care of their own patients within the hospital and not involving themselves in something that they believe has no direct, immediate concern to the practice of psychiatry.

As an initial step in breaking down the dichotomy between the institutional *us* and the community *them,* the administrator should give his *personal* attention to any activity that involves the community coming into the hospital. Whenever possible, he should meet with community groups or even with an individual who would like to undertake an enterprise in connection with the institution. In dealing with community groups, the adminstrator should take a positive attitude, rather than insist that the community group immediately concern itself with all the possible problems and dangers of a new program. Nothing is so destructive to an enthusiastic but inexperienced outsider as to be questioned in a suspicious manner about all the details of his plan. Nor can the administrator set prematurely sharp boundaries around what is suitable activity and what is not. For example, a community group might suggest that it utilize an emptied hospital building as a settlement house, with the idea of providing a therapeutic atmosphere for its difficult young people, and perhaps improving relations between the hospital and the community. Whether this is in fact a good idea will depend on many circumstances. Our point here is to emphasize how important it is for the administrator to have an open mind about such new possibilities, which may have an eventual payoff for his more immediate related problems: for example, local youth destroying hospital property or the community's view of the hospital as something alien, full of frightening people.

In an institution's relations with the community in general, and especially with a group that becomes involved in a basically local activity, it is important that the administrator not get embroiled in issues of power and control. This is worth stressing, particularly if the institution is in an urban, lower-class setting, but it is equally true in working with any community group. The most vital kind of community engagement is likely to come from eager, involved, sometimes rebellious people who like to feel they are participating in decision-making and are not just being used as handmaidens or money raisers. If an administrator shows his readiness to listen to whatever grievances—founded or unfounded —they may have had against the institution in the past and to cooperate with them, they in turn will be able to acknowledge their own areas of ignorance and to recognize their sometimes unreasonable requests. It is true that such an attitude on the part of the administrator does not preclude some controversies and problematic issues about power and authority. However, if the attitude prevails that all participants are concerned with getting the job done and that all can work together collaboratively, the issue of who is the boss is less likely to be a stumbling block. In short, our philosophy in working with the community is the same as in working inside the institution. We try to promote creativity and flexibility and to encourage people to get away from rigid, hierarchical modes of functioning.

It is consistent with this philosophy that the administrator's position was to support a diversity of efforts and orientations on the part of the community. The same pluralism that was part of the philosophy regarding the staff's treatment of patients (to be described in the next chapter) also applied to the community's efforts within the hospital. For example, the new administration welcomed many different kinds of volunteers, each group with its own ideas on how best to help the hospital. They ranged from middle-aged women who liked to bring food to hospital functions, through case aides who, under supervison, had intensive one-to-one relationships, to bearded college students who showed psychedelic movies on the chronic wards.

The same kind of diversity was promoted for all kinds of efforts to break down the barriers between hospital and community. We helped one psychiatric resident raise money to carry out a plan to take long-term schizophrenic men and women out to visit former patients who had been abandoned by their families and who now resided in nursing homes for the elderly.[3] One unit held a multiagency conference about a day hospital patient with myriad economic, familial, and intrapsychic problems. A point was made to include in our guest lecture series speakers who were concerned with community problems and the relationship between the hospital and the community. With the assistance of the Northern New England Branch of the American Psychiatric Association, we arranged to have a conference on poverty and mental illness held on the grounds of the hospital.[4] Posters and letters emphasized that the conference was open to staff of all levels and to paraprofessional groups of all interests.

These and other activities served to educate staff about their role in the community and the community's role in the hospital. Staff members were amazed, for example, to discover the great number of people and agencies involved in the case of the day hospital patient mentioned above. The conference on poverty and mental illness served to highlight for staff the interrelationship between poverty and a whole host of social disorders, including mental illness.

Holding such a conference may seem removed from the problem of educating staff to accept the community's entering the hospital or to go out into the community. But changes in behavior are often preceded by changes in orientation and thinking. As the staff member realizes, for example, that the slum may be his worst enemy in terms of creating new cases of mental illness or of raising the readmissions of discharged patients, he will be more prepared to view consulting to a settlement house as part of his professional identity. Seeing these interrelations and meeting face to face the various agencies and people involved can help the staff member and the community worker view their problems as joint ones. This kind of sharing can do much to end a game in which no one, least of all the patient, wins: a game of *us* and *them* in which the social agency blames the hospital for discharging a patient too early and the hospital blames *them* for "dumping" a patient on *us*.

Another important task is to educate staff to take a long-term view of community-hospital relations. It is true, for example, that initially outsiders on a ward can be upsetting to staff and patients. However, in the long run, the benefits far outweigh the temporary discomfiture since it is only through such additional, unpaid help that the patients can get much of the attention they need. Staff's objections that their service needs limit the time they can give to community involvement have a sharp validity, but only on a short-term basis. The administrator should help them realize that ultimately community groups can yield a bigger payoff by providing care for discharged patients and by anticipating and managing crises that would have returned patients to the hospital.

As a matter of administrative principle, staff members who are able to knock down the barriers between *us* and *them* should be rewarded in some tangible way. An institution that puts a high priority on strong community relations should give special recognition to those who possess some of the qualities needed in this area—energy, warmth, a relatively egalitarian manner, and a willingness to enter uncharted areas where questions are many and clear answers few.

Institutions of Learning

It would be difficult to overestimate for any hospital the value of contacts with institutions of higher learning. Universities can bring to a state hospital particularly a quest for new ideas and new approaches that can help break down the hospital's intellectual isolation and obsession with the usual ways of doing things. They also have resources of people and money which, in addition to whatever long-term contribution they may make to the practice of psychiatry, have an immediate effect on the hospital (a value that cannot be ignored). For example, a clinical study of a given group of patients may not only help the students in their search for new methods of treatment, but it may also have a direct service benefit by giving the patients additional attention.

Unfortunately, close relationships between state hospitals and institutions of higher learning are by and large not fully developed. One stumbling block is often the attitude of hospital staff. Some staff members are reluctant to permit students to enter their bailiwicks for fear that these outsiders will not understand their way of doing things, will be overcritical, will eat up too much of their time, and so forth. Others resent the students' leisurely way of pursuing their goals, especially when they themselves are overburdened with work, constantly harassed by the pressure of time.

The administrator committed to the importance of bringing graduate students into the hospital or other institutions such as schools, government agencies, and the like, must help staff see their value. To counteract staff's fear of criticism, perhaps the greatest reason for their resistance, the new administrator early in his tenure would do well to set an example by permitting students to observe and evaluate his own activities. Of course he takes the risk of being criticized; alert students are always critical. But he shows staff that he is not asking them to do something he is not himself doing. If he reacts to these criticisms with neither angry defensiveness nor overwhelming guilt, he communicates several important messages: that it is not so dangerous to be criticized; that confrontation with one's own image, although painful at first, can be an invaluable asset in improving one's functioning; and, most important of all, that the students' observations can often provide a formula for planning favorable change.

Another general policy is to urge staff to invest a portion of their time in teaching. Boston State particularly encouraged any educational innovations or extensions of the training program to groups that had hitherto not been included. For example, several staff members arranged an elective course at the hospital for first-year medical students. (Prior to this, the education of medical students at the hospital had been confined to those in their third and fourth years.) The new course was not limited to the traditional diagnosis, evaluation, and short-term treatment of the patient, but included the student's becoming familiar with both the ward and the family life of the patient.

Although opening of the institution to educational centers is the first major step, it is by no means sufficient in itself. The long years of estrangement mean that the university does not automatically think of the state hospital, or for that matter other urban public organizations, as a training site, and may not even be aware of changed conditions that would make it more attractive for academic use. In addition, many university departments concentrate their academic teaching in small centers, which are identified as their specific teaching hospitals. Just as the state hospital is often seen as a second-rate place for patient treatment when compared with a small center, so it is also seen as a second-rate place for learning, to be used, if at all, as a choice of last resort.

This image can be changed if the administrator makes active efforts to point out all the advantages of a state hospital as a training center. One of the greatest advantages lies in its size. Because a state hospital has a large patient census, it has possibilities for the student that do not exist elsewhere. Often, small university centers are so crowded with educational and research programs that the patients' appointment books contain a more crammed schedule than those of staff members. Students frequently complain that there is not enough clinical material to go around, and the fights for patients can be destructive to morale. Enterprising teachers and students often welcome an educational setting such as that of the open state hospital where programs can be developed side by side without treading on one another's toes. Also, state hospitals are less likely to be overprotective, to worry about "what is being done to the patients," thus giving students more freedom to experiment with new approaches.

Another advantage is the great wealth and diversity of clinical material. At a state hospital, the student can see the full range of mental and social deviance—acute and chronic schizophrenia, drug addiction, criminality, alcoholism, problems of the aged as well as those of the adolescent, and so on. What so often is a burden to staff and what appears so frightening to the average layman can be converted into a rich learning experience for the resourceful student.

Two other advantages that a large state hospital can offer should not be ignored or treated casually, even though they may seem on the surface to be relatively minor. One is the large, open land area, which makes parking free and easy. Quick accessibility to a training center is a plus value in recruiting a busy teacher or a student with a crowded schedule. The second is the availability of space within buildings that can be easily converted into offices, classrooms, and laboratories. This is no small matter to academicians, who need both privacy and adequate room to work properly.

Granted that the administrator has made staff receptive to students entering the hospital, and that he has stimulated interest in the state hospital as a training site, what further considerations should he bear in mind? What further steps should he take?

Depending on its nearness to a large city, of course, the most desirable situation would be to set up associations with as many schools as possible. Since a state hospital does not usually have an exclusive arrangement with any one college or university, it is possible to affiliate with many, depending on interests, staff affinities, and resources. If it is to establish multiple connections, the hospital must show considerable flexibility in the kinds of relationships it develops with different departments and different schools. Sometimes it is one in which a hospital staff member provides clinical field instruction for students of, say, psychology, with the staff member having a joint appointment at both the hospital and the university. In other instances, a staff member may have a quite informal relationship with students interested in learning about his particular area of investigation. In still other instances, an instructor primarily located outside the hospital may come in to teach his specialty to the hospital staff.

We would emphasize that, in the developing phase, it is wise for the hospital to begin an informal connection with a local university and then move to a more formal contractual arrangement after the benefits of the collaboration have been tangibly perceived by both sides. If one waits for all official clearances to be obtained before, for example, a special course is fully approved by the university, one can get bogged down in endless delays.

By working in a variety of ways at Boston State, we were able to expand or establish university affiliations with many departments at Tufts, Harvard, Boston, Brandeis, and Northeastern universities, the Massachusetts Institute of Technology, Simmons College, and the University of Massachusetts. Students coming to the hospital included not only those from schools of medicine and nursing, but also from departments of psychology, sociology, social work, physical education, theology, rehabilitation, public relations, and occupational therapy. The hospital also provided training experience for students from Harvard's Laboratory of Community Psychiatry and the Law-Medicine Institute of Boston University. By a complementary arrangement, our own staff members were permitted to participate in courses that were normally open only to students formally enrolled at the school.

Once again, it is essential that the administrator realize the importance of personal relations in developing this area, as he has others. If he has helped to facilitate the research or educational program of a local university by opening the hospital's doors, allaying staff suspicion, and seeing that much of the detail work gets done so that the right people are in touch with each other, he has simultaneously set the stage for someone at the university reciprocating when the hospital needs access to the school's facilities. Sometimes, out of negotiations over a very modest first step in collaboration, for example, a joint program of study for one student, can grow a major educational or research collaboration between the two institutions.

Today's administrators of our urban service organizations have the optimum historical moment to move toward a much closer collaboration between their institutions and local universities. Students of all disciplines are crying for closer contact with the real problems of the world, especially those that concern the economically deprived and socially neglected members of our community. They also want to acquire this learning not in some overprotected, oversupervised, ivory-tower atmosphere, but in a climate that gives them some elbow room and a chance to experiment. A bold administrator can join forces with bold students in innovating all kinds of educational programs that could have considerable service implications at the immediate level and even greater implications for the future.

Public Relations

In a sense it is gratuitous to have a separate section on public relations since we have been discussing it implicitly, if not explicitly, throughout this chapter. If there is favorable change in the hospital structure, then patients and staff will have a more positive image of the institution and their role in it. If the barriers are broken down between the hospital and the academic community, then universities will not see the institution as barren, devoid of intellectual activity. If citizens are involved with hospital programs, they will be less likely to stigmatize the discharged mental patient as incapable of assuming a responsible, decent role in society.

If we have been reluctant to stress public relations per se, there is a very valid reason. To most psychiatrists, the very concept of public relations is anathema. It smacks of Madison Avenue, over-selling, overpromising. Furthermore, it is contrary to the whole mystique of psychotherapy, which takes place in an atmosphere of anonymity and quiet.

It is our contention, however, that despite psychiatrists' negative feelings about public relations, the administrator of a large mental hospital must be concerned with his hospital's image. Moreover, if he is to do the job properly, he needs the assistance of skilled persons specially trained in this area. As things stand at present, in most state hospitals and other public institutions, the day-to-day public relations activities, for example, distribution of stories to press and arranging tours for guests, are handled in a piecemeal, uncoordinated fashion by various staff members, with the administrator or his secretary frequently shouldering the burden. No private industry the size of our large state hospitals would or could manage its public relations in this haphazard manner. Yet this is what usually happens in an area where we are dealing with the most sensitive of all issues—mental illness—and with a public that is prepared to believe the worst about our efforts.

An important part of the public relations operation in a large institution is to keep both the staff and the outside community up to date about its progress. Too often, there is a time lag between the changes that have occurred and knowledge of these improvements. Without some kind of concerted effort on the part of the hospital staff, the average person's image of the institution remains fixed on an earlier reality or seizes only those elements in the present that correspond with the record of the past, frequently overlooking favorable developments.

Our last point calls attention to the importance not only of correcting misconceptions, but also of setting accurate perceptions in a proper context. For example, when outside people visit an institution and are not simply given a Russian tour of the best facilities, but are taken everywhere, they are likely to be shocked by the conditions that still exist in many of its buildings. Those concerned with public relations have the particular responsibility of pointing out areas where some progress has been achieved, particularly those in which the best developed from what was once a very deplorable situation. It both interests and instructs people more to see a *development* than to see either the very good or the very bad.

It is also part of public relations to convey this same sense of perspective to staff. If personnel complain, for example, of the low staff-patient ratio, it is important to point out that conditions were much worse a few years back and that, at the present rate of change, they should be considerably better in the near future. Of course, staff should not be informed of improvements in a way that suggests that "you never had it so good," or that the institution is on the verge of instant utopia. But they should be helped to see what has been done despite the problems that still remain.

Although complaints from staff and community are painful to hear, they may be indicative of an overall state of improvement in public relations. As we know from other kinds of social change, demands and complaints are most likely to appear in a climate of rising expectations, rather than at times when conditions are at their worst. The most difficult task in public relations, either external or internal, is dealing with silent, hopeless apathy. It is much better for the public to criticize the institution than to be indifferent.

Sometimes these criticisms are brought to the attention of the mass media and reported as an exposé. This brings us to the complex question of whether the administration can utilize negative publicity in a positive way. One position would be that this sequence is very much in line with the American tradition. If a bad condition exists, expose it to the light of publicity, and it will be changed. Get the people stirred up and start a crusade. Unfortunately, matters are not so simple. The public's interest is often fickle, and the real issues of today's scandal are forgotten by tomorrow, leaving the average citizen with a vague feeling that the publicized institution is a terrible one and "somebody should do something about it." This is not to imply that the administrator should go out of his way to avoid a bad press by "running scared," looking into every conceivable matter that one day might erupt into a cause célèbre. It does mean that if such a situation does occur, he should meet it aggressively, not taking a defensive stand, but focusing his efforts on the real issues.

Some of the issues concerning negative publicity are illustrated by the following incident, which occurred a year after our arrival at Boston State. A newly elected, aggressive, welfare-minded young legislator had heard that living conditions were deplorable in one of our buildings. He requested a tour of the hospital, and was conducted around by a staff member, who had been instructed to show him anything he wanted to see, particularly the deficiences and inadequacies he was looking for. The legislator then asked about forty colleagues to join him in a return visit, this time with the press in attendance. The result was distressingly negative publicity, pointing the finger of blame at the hospital administration and the department of mental health. The Massachusetts Association for Mental Health, through their own channels, helped interpret the deficiences as essentially related to an inadequate hospital budget, turning the finger of scorn back on the legislators. The department of mental health indicated that the legislature had failed to pass the superintendent's request for 273 new positions, which had been approved by the department. Soon a newspaper editorial appeared, putting matters in a more honest perspective. This stimulated other newspaper stories, which reported positive gains made by the hospital staff despite the serious shortages.

Whatever stress and lingering negative effects this episode had, it also contained some positive features. Some legislators did get to know more about conditions at the hospital. It did give the Massachusetts Association for Mental Health an opportunity to rally to our support and point out the need for better care of the mentally ill everywhere. The community did have an opportunity to learn about the measures being taken to correct some defects of the hospital. Indeed, it is only through publicity of one kind or another that the community can learn where its monies are being spent well or where the internal structure and leadership of an institution are so ineffective that money alone can be of little help. It also acquainted staff with some of the hubbub and upset that inevitably accompany the growing pains of a closer relationship between the hospital and the community.

The incident with the legislators highlights the importance of a state hospital having an office specifically devoted to public relations. A large mental hospital is always sitting on a keg of dynamite. Even though there may in fact be proportionally fewer acts of violence committed by mental patients than by persons outside, every such occurrence is likely to set off a wave of publicity and far more public outrage than if the act were committed by a so-called normal person. A skilled public relations professional is needed to provide the news media with the correct background information quickly, to coordinate staff reactions, and to make sure misrepresentations are immediately refuted. More than that, a good public relations expert knows when *not* to make an issue.

Consistent with this viewpoint, we set up a public relations department at Boston State. We found that the usefulness of a good public relations officer is not limited to the handling of crises. As a regular undertaking, apart from sending out releases to the news media, he can do much to build up staff morale, even by such simple innovations as a staff newsletter or a comprehensive hospital telephone directory. He can arrange meetings, make visitors' trips informative and fruitful, coordinate staff publications, and prepare brochures. He can certainly help develop everyone's awareness of the hospital's progress as well as its problems. If he has discretion and taste, the sine qua non of a good public relations officer, he never needs to oversell, but just to "tell it like it is."

As important as a public relations department is, it must work in very close collaboration with the hospital leadership. We simply have to find new ways to get the hospital message across to the public honestly and constructively. Whatever the many determinants of our reticence and our wish for obscurity, they are no longer tenable in view of the huge demands facing the mental health profession. A state hospital is loaded with human drama which must be conveyed in a way that challenges the public to help with the task. However great our personal efforts with individuals, or even groups of citizens, we can never really accomplish our goals if we do not utilize the tremendous potential of the mass media for education, stimulation, and involvement.

REFERENCES

1. E. Goffman, *Asylums* (New York: Doubleday-Anchor, 1961).

2. I. Belknap, *Human Problems of a State Mental Hospital* (New York: McGraw-Hill, 1956); A. Deutsch, *The Mentally Ill in America*, 2nd ed. (New York: Columbia University Press, 1949); M. Greenblatt, D. J. Levin-

son, and R. H. Williams, eds., *The Patient and the Mental Hospital* (Glencoe: Free Press, 1957); and M. J. Ward, *The Snake Pit* (New York: Random House, 1946).

3. Jerome Collins, "Patient Helping Patient," *Hospital and Community Psychiatry* 18 (1967): 239–42.

4. M. Greenblatt, P. E. Emery, and B. C. Glueck, Jr., eds., *Poverty and Mental Health*, Psychiatry Research Report 21 (Washington: American Psychiatric Association, 1967).

CHAPTER 3

Philosophy of Treatment: Some Issues and Difficulties

Aside from our reference to the community aspects of the hospital's overall program, we have not discussed treatment ideology in general or at Boston State in particular. This is of primary importance, since a psychiatric hospital is frequently known for the particular kind of treatment it favors, which is usually a reflection of the orientation of its administrator.

Whatever treatment philosophy a new administrator espouses, he should make his predilections known to staff early. This does not mean that he must rush with his decision; nor does it mean he cannot modify it as time goes on. But it is important, especially in a state hospital, with its tendency toward stagnation and inertia, that the superintendent present as early as possible some kind of rallying point and sense of direction to the hospital community. A state hospital—like many urban service organizations—is so imbued with a negative character that constant, conscious efforts must be made to create a positive identity, an important component of which is the kinds of philosophy—therapeutic, educational, rehabilitative—it emphasizes.

Another advantage of the new administrator's stating his philosophy early is that he is likely to command more sharp public attention at the beginning of his regime than at any other time during his tenure. Staff as well as the outside professional community are very keen and indeed anxious to know what the new man believes in, what he stands for, what fields he is going to push, and where he is going to take the institution.

Whatever decision about treatment the new administrator makes will necessarily have its costs and gains, but the very act of making it communicates to all that a particular philosophy has been formulated. If he balks or temporizes, the administrator has communicated something else: that he is the kind of leader who responds more to the interests and preferences of others and will not be a source of clear direction himself. This does not mean that all new ideas must come from the top man. On the contrary, a resourceful leader is always ready to utilize the ideas of others and to broadcast the source of the inspiration. However, he assimilates these ideas so that they form part of his philosophy and gives them the kind of enthusiasm and push that must be supplied if they are to be concretely implemented.

When the going gets rough, subordinates expect their leader to make the final decisions regarding priorities in the distribution of resources, personnel, and so on. These choices in turn are very much influenced by the leader's treatment philosophy. If he has not clearly worked out what he wishes the hospital to stand for, he is in danger of being pushed around by the most powerful lobby or group inside or outside the hospital. In this atmosphere, his decisions about priorities are likely to be seen as impulsive reactions to pressures around him rather than as considered steps in a total program development that reflects an overall philosophical direction. When he behaves in this fashion, he is —to paraphrase Napoleon—permitting events to dictate policy rather than policy to dictate events.

Thus, the new administrator will find that the making of important decisions about treatment philosophies is not a one-time thing, but requires continual reaffirmation in the face of pressure and demands that they be changed or drastically modified.

As we shall see, a decision about the basic philosophy of treatment usually contains a number of other implicit or explicit decisions about other competing treatments, about which staff members are best equipped to carry out the preferred modes of treatment, and about what kinds of patients respond best to the kinds of treatment the hospital is committed to pursue.

An Eclectic Approach Versus a Single System

A primary decision that a new administrator must make is whether he is going to foster multiple treatment modalities or a single unified framework. This is a particularly crucial choice since it carries with it serious consequences for all aspects of the hospital's functioning.

Some hospital administrators choose a single framework, for example, the psychodynamic ideology, as a unifying framework. In such an institution, one will find a great concentration on one-to-one intensive psychotherapy. The theory is that the essential impasses to a patient's functioning are intrapsychic and that these internal conflicts can only be worked through in a transference relationship within which the patient reexperiences earlier conflicts, gains insight into their origins, and learns, after painful introspection, to function more appropriately.

In many institutions, particularly small university-affiliated hospitals, this preference for psychotherapy is seen as part of an overall hierarchy of treatments. Psychotherapy is at the top because it promises the greatest benefit to the patient and requires, presumably, a sensitive, skilled, and experienced therapist. Of all treatment modalities, it is viewed as both the core of the young psychiatrist's education and the most difficult skill to learn. Group therapy and family therapy may also be highly valued, but they are often seen as a less intensive treatment form.

In such a hierarchy, milieu therapy is clearly considered as less prestigious than the preceding treatments. The view is that initially the milieu provides a kind of benign envelope within which the patient resides while the "real work" is being done in psychotherapy. Milieu activity, such as work therapy, is thought of as something the patient can truly benefit from only after progress is made in psychotherapy. Milieu therapy is also regarded as something the young mental health worker can learn by doing, in contrast to the more favored treatment forms, which must be carefully supervised. Lowest in rank is pharmacotherapy. Psychotropic drugs are regarded as only temporary palliatives for patients to make them accessible to more preferred treatment modalities. Psychopharmacotherapy is also seen as something relatively easy for the student to learn.

Implicit in this kind of hierarchy is a matching hierarchy of personnel. Since psychotherapy is the most valuable form of treatment and the most difficult to learn, the belief is that its practice should be limited to psychiatrists, although meritorious psychologists and social workers are sometimes permitted to join the club. Because milieu therapy requires good human qualities but no refined skills, its practice can be left to a wide variety of ancillary personnel under appropriate psychiatric leadership. Pharmacotherapy is a bit paradoxical—its medical nature clearly requires the sanction of a physician, but because of its lackluster appeal, the actual impetus for prescribing drugs is often left to someone low on the personnel hierarchy.

In contrast, when social or milieu therapy is the predominant modality, the daily life of the patient and the total hospital environment are utilized as the main vehicles for treatment. Individual psychotherapy is likely to be downgraded since it is seen as working against the open group spirit of the place, although this treatment may be available for the instruction of interested students. Psychopharmaceuticals are again regarded as secondary to the group process of treatment, grudgingly used in emergencies. With this kind of hierarchy of treatment, the hierarchy of personnel is also very different from that of a psychoanalytically oriented institution. There is emphasis on equality, role diffusion, and on "everyone being therapeutic." Indeed, there is some tendency for an absolute reversal of the traditional hierarchy, with patients and aides being regarded as the most effective treatment agents, since they are closest to the real life situation and with it the longest. In such social therapeutic institutions as Synanon, for example, professionals may be viewed with suspicion, if indeed not completely prohibited.

It must be said that there are certain clear advantages to having a unified framework, of whatever kind it may be. Obviously, one treatment form can be pushed more effectively if all resources and attention support it, rather than being spread out over several modalities. If part of the efficacy of the treatment seems to reside in the enthusiasm with which that therapy is dispensed, such enthusiasm is likely to be stronger where one tone pervades the entire institution, rather than the cacaphony of controversy that occurs when strong-minded proponents of different treatment ideologies coexist under the same roof. A single system may inspire students with a sense of structure and purpose in the complex directions of psychiatric endeavor, which are often so confusing and discouraging to the novice. A single system can also help the administrator weld together a group of like-minded people and so help diminish some of the difficulties of running a large, heterogeneous organization. If he clearly announces when he takes over that he is for *X*, proponents of *Y* will realize this is not the place for them and leave, permitting him to make replacements with *X* adherents. This same process will occur in the self-selection that goes on in terms of recruitment: *X* adherents will come to the institution and *X* doubters or opponents won't even bother to apply.

Despite the many advantages of a single framework, the administrator's position at Boston State was to reject this concept. His decision in favor of multiple treatment forms reflected in part his own temperament and personality. But it also reflected very strong theoretical convictions. The idea of a single conceptual framework, along *whatever* lines, is not appropriate to the present stage of development of psychiatric knowledge. No single ideological position can possibly serve either to guide our future adequately in view of our massive ignorance about the etiology and disease process of mental illness or to encompass the advances that have been made in other fields, such as biology, sociology, and education. As a teaching model, a single position narrows the student's gaze unduly, hinders his intellectual development, and rigidifies speculation and possibilities into dogma. It reduces his tolerance of the "welter of complexities," to use Alfred North Whitehead's term, and shields him from the increasing ambiguities of contemporary psychiatry.

Most important perhaps are the implications for practical service. Whatever gains there might be to patients through the messianic fervor of a one-treatment institution, they are more than offset by the inevitable exclusion of other treatments. This consideration carries particular force at a state hospital with its wide diversity of patients and the community's mandate that the hospital accept all who wish to be admitted whether they fit the administrator's preferred treatment form or not. For example, the state hospital superintendent cannot accept only young, well-educated, middle-class patients because they seem to respond best to psychotherapy. Furthermore, with its heavy admission load, a state hospital cannot stress individual long-term therapy without doing considerable injustice to patients who are deemed unsuitable for this treatment or who are precluded from it because of shortage of staff.

The same oversimplification of psychiatric complexities that occurs when individual psychodynamics are the sole center of focus also occurs when any of the other therapies is put at the top of the treatment ladder. A sole emphasis on milieu therapy would be detrimental to those patients who might be especially responsive to psychotherapy or somatic therapy. It also seemed to us as unreasonable to deny students the opportunity to learn about these treatment forms as it was to make one or another of them the sole learning experience.

Finally, if one of the objectives in the reorganization of Boston State was to motivate the creative potential of all personnel, achieving this goal would be hindered by a treatment hierarchy that implicitly or explicitly favored one occupational group over another. Nonmedical personnel must not feel "ancillary" to psychiatrists, as would be the case if psychotherapy ruled the scene. Nor should professionals feel that they could not pursue specialities of their own interests. People, not psychotropic drugs, were to be the main sources of therapeutic hope, but neither was vigorous pursuit of what the somatic therapies could in fact accomplish to be excluded.

In short, the administrator communicated to staff very soon his decision in favor of a multiple treatment approach. This was not expressed simply as a laissez-faire tolerance of varying viewpoints, but as an active and firm commitment to the principle of diversity. He encouraged the introduction of new ideas, advocated by enthusiastic representatives of different points of view, from such diverse groups as students, volunteers, and senior psychiatrists. He also encouraged the establishment of demonstration and training programs, pushing in a variety of directions.

To implement the decision for multiple directions, a program of social psychiatry was added to the already ongoing vigorous program in the psychotherapy of psychoses. Seminars in neurology and neuropathology were strengthened. Programs in rehabilitation were stepped up. Drug therapy became an important competitive modality. Training in family therapy was expanded, and continuing efforts were made to develop milieu programs. The points of view of community psychiatry were constantly promoted by a growing cadre of professionals working outside the hospital.

The administrator also communicated to the medical public that Boston State was a place in which reasonable new ideas would be given a fair trial. This was done with the hope of attracting people with creative gifts, some of whom had heretofore been labeled as "way-out" by their more conventional colleagues. The conviction was that much progress could be made by those who were regarded as radical or even bizarre. Furthermore, administration wanted to prevent any comfortable settling down into a conventional eclectic program, where diversity was accepted, but only along known, traditional lines. We hoped that the hospital would always remain open to a new idea, no matter how outlandish it might initially seem. This approach was in keeping with the basic conviction that what was known in psychiatry was but a grain of sand on the vast beaches of the unknown. No narrow pride or professional chauvinism should lead us to prejudge the worthiness of an idea.

In short, Boston State began to be known not for one treatment philosophy but for its aggressive multiple endeavors and its receptivity to new ideas. This had distinct advantages in attracting able young staff who knew that they would be given the opportunity not only to present their innovative plans, but also to implement them pragmatically. This approach can be applied at other larger public institutions that face formidable competition, indeed often overwhelming competition, from smaller centers. Higher salaries alone will not attract able talent; the most powerful incentive is the freedom of staff to try new concepts and techniques.

Although Boston State undoubtedly lost out on students who wished to train at an institution that featured their particular interest—and this was usually psychotherapy—we were able to attract those who wanted exposure to the full gamut of psychiatric treatments and techniques. In this connection, we were very fortunate in that the administrator's own interest corresponded to a shift of direction in American psychiatry. During the 1950s, most students were predominantly interested in learning psychodynamics, and it was clearly the most prestigious area of endeavor. By the 1960s, there was a growing realization, especially among students, that new approaches were needed and that few final answers had been found.

From a service point of view, an argument could doubtless be made that a full commitment to a unified treatment program that was suitable for state hospital patients, for example, milieu therapy or behavior therapy, would have had real advantages. But to do this would have severely limited the training and research thrust of the institution. It would, in the long run, have hindered service by decreasing the total amount of stimulation, people, and resources.

Although an assertive multiple-treatment approach had distinct advantages, it created its own problems. Many key people at the hospital were committed to the more unified psychotherapeutic framework, which had dominated major divisions of the institution for some time. They were bound to be critical, and indeed many of them were, of a movement in a more eclectic direction. However, they were not as antagonistic as they would have been had we tried to direct the hospital toward a single, unified treatment approach in a modality other than that of their own preferences. They were able to continue doing "their thing," even though they were acutely unhappy about some of the things others were doing.

We found that a philosophy of diversity means that an administrator must be able to tolerate key people who may not share his enthusiasm for multiple approaches. Indeed, there are distinct advantages that not everybody in an eclectic institution be themselves eclectic in interest. We mentioned earlier that treatment is often more effective when administered by a "true believer." To some extent, an eclectic institution can maintain some of this single-minded enthusiasm by having units where the leaders are free to push on in their own directions. The top administrator must steer a delicate course to avoid undermining their enthusiasm, but at the same time he must insist that others have the same freedom they have. In such an eclectic institution, people are free to pursue what they love, but they are not free to stop others from having the same privilege.

Thus, the administrator of a multiple-treatment institution must be alert to the ambitions of proponents of one or another philosophy who wish not only to expand their own empires but also to limit the efforts of those with whom they disagree. For example, a senior figure committed to carefully supervised psychotherapy may become outraged at a program that features behavior therapy or the use of volunteers for intensive work with patients. The administrator must be prepared to arbitrate such controversies among his staff members, all the while protecting the principle of diversity.

As a matter of fact, a philosophy of diversity poses severe challenges to the administrator. It can easily degenerate into a kind of therapeutic nihilism or a frenzied exchange of polemics. It can also slowly give ground to one or another powerful group pushing its own unified framework. The administrator must be prepared for the criticism that in his eclecticism he really stands for nothing, only a piecemeal, unsynthesized accretion of ideas and programs. But, the administrator of a multiple-treatment institution at its best can find heartening the knowledge that he has not arbitrarily excluded any possible help for patients, that he has helped to expose students to the full range of theories, practices, and career directions, and that he has kept the doors open to new knowledge.

Dealing with Community Opposition to Treatment Policy

Decisions concerning treatment philosophy are often very difficult to make, but once made they usually do not involve dramatic repercussions from the public that sorely test the administrator's commitment to his ideas. True, when a program that utilizes paramedical personnel as primary therapists is used, a relative may be upset that a case aide rather than a physician is taking care of the patient and will complain directly to the administrator. But, in most instances, the public is inclined to trust the judgment of the hospital. Moreover, if there *is* dissatisfaction with treatment, it is not likely to take an organized form.

By way of contrast, we now wish to discuss an institutional decision—the open-door policy—that was relatively easy to make, but extremely difficult to maintain in the face of organized opposition from the community.

It is not necessary to review here the many arguments in favor of an open-door hospital, that is, one with as few locked wards as possible. It is sufficient to say that on the whole our administration favored such a policy, although it recognized that the policy could not become a dogma and that there were undoubtedly some patients who did require a confined setting. This did not alter the position that in many gray instances the administrator preferred to take some of the risks of openness rather than move in the direction of confinement and restraint.

Initially, the task at Boston State was not so much to make this decision as it was to continue Dr. Barton's pioneering commitment to an open institution. However, it is an extremely challenging problem for an administrator to maintain an open hospital in an urban environment, with its increasing concern about violence and crime. Since no hospital can be absolutely perfect in its diagnosis of which patients will commit dangerous acts if given some freedom, the administrator committed to relative openness must be prepared to stand by his decision despite community pressure that he accede to its demands for locked doors. He personally must be prepared to maintain a very exposed position. The criticism will be far worse if a patient given some freedom commits a violent act than if a patient commits such an act after escaping through barriers to freedom. Also, one act of violence has greater significance to the public than the many instances of patients who have benefited from the relative freedom of the hospital.

These problems can be seen in more concrete form by considering a specific instance and its aftermath.

A young man was sent to the hospital by the court for psychiatric evaluation after being arrested for accosting a woman sexually. Several days before his case was to be tried in court, he failed to show up for work at the hospital cafeteria, left the grounds, and broke into a house nearby, where he attempted to rape a young woman. Fortunately her mother heard her cries, forced her way into the room, and fought off the intruder. The patient escaped and returned quickly to the ward, where he confessed everything to his favorite attendant.

The legal and psychiatric complexities of the case are too numerous to take up here. Suffice it to say that this terrible incident was responsible for a very considerable storm, bringing together in confrontation both the outside community and representatives of the hospital.

Local newspapers printed the story of the attempted rape and editorialized about the crime committed by this "court case." Friends and neighbors of the young woman, together with other anxious citizens, were up in arms against the hospital. They pleaded for action from their local state legislators, who, in response, demanded a meeting with the superintendent. At what turned out to be a passionate encounter, the citizens and the legislators vociferated against a possible repetition of this grave incident. They also gave full expression to a gamut of irritations and humiliations they had endured over the years, together with their anxieties about living near a mental hospital.

The complaints spilled out rapidly: patients were allowed to roam at will in the streets and shops near the hospital; they were badly clothed and their appearance was often bizarre; they were a menace to motorists since they appeared to be oblivious to the flow of traffic. Complaints came from mothers: some patients either stared menacingly at their children or threatened them with vile language. One timid, elderly woman confessed, almost in tears, that some male patients had used her garden as a urinal. A store owner asked who was going to pay for the pilferage from her grocery counters. Property owners were the most vocal: the patients' presence on the streets impaired the value of their dwellings and made rentals difficult.

The foregoing is just a distillate of the many outcries against the hospital administration. After all were given as much time as they wanted to complain, they were asked what measures they could recommend to alleviate the problems. We shall list but a few:

1. The hospital should be moved to a rural area since it was improperly located in what had become an urban community.

2. The doors to *all* hospital wards and buildings should be locked.

3. The doors on those wards where court cases resided should be locked.

4. Sentinels should be stationed at the gates, checking on patient privileges, making certain no patient leaves the grounds unless he has been given permission to do so.

5. Patients should be intensively screened at the ward level and no one allowed out whose habits and deportment are unacceptable to the community.

6. The legislature should at once greatly increase the complement of hospital police, especially those on the night force. An alternative was to request the Boston police to make twenty-four hour rounds of the hospital area.

7. Maximum security wards should be set up immediately on the hospital grounds, and in other state hospitals as well.

8. A legislative committee should investigate the handling of mental patients who are security risks.

Obviously, the philosophy espoused by the community was in sharp opposition to the open-door policy of the hospital. Indeed, triggered by the extremely dangerous incident just described, many long-standing grievances were dredged up. Administration had to recognize that what we took for granted was not at all taken as a matter of course by the community. We also had to recognize that we had failed to convince them of the therapeutic values of an open hospital and had not helped them sufficiently with the inevitable problems such a policy presents.

Our failing in this regard is a common one. Too often, mental health workers assume that others are imbued with the same overall ideological attitudes toward the mentally ill. We forget that the average person in the community is neither trained nor paid to take an understanding view of mental illness. As the authors of *Action for Mental Health* point out,[1] mentally ill persons are often very disturbing in their behavior and in a way that provokes others to dislike and to reject them.

It should not come as any surprise that people in the community are upset, or even outraged, if their children are exposed to vile language, if their shops are pilfered, if their property is devalued. We must also remember that until about twenty years ago, a custodial attitude toward the mentally ill pervaded the thinking of not only the general public, but the psychiatric profession as well. One cannot erase in two decades the public's deeply engrained point of view that mental patients should be hidden out of sight and that the community should be carefully protected from them.

What, then, should the hospital administrator do when his open-door policy is directly challenged by the community, partly because of real grievances and partly because of long-standing custodial attitudes? If he really meets their demands, he will inevitably violate the rights of patients; that is, he cannot restrict all potential "disturbers of the peace" without also restricting many who would be unlikely to bother anyone. If he were to place all "risky" patients on locked wards, he would deprive them of the benefits that come from mingling with better adjusted patients. Moreover, a definition of "risky" that would satisfy the community might very well mean locking up a huge number of patients. Although such a policy may assuage the public, it would not truly meet their objections. Short of building maximum security sections, a locked ward in itself does not prevent a determined patient from leaving the hospital.

Could not "risky" patients be sent to a maximum security facility for the criminally insane? Such facilities—in Massachusetts, as well as in most states—are nowhere near adequate to handle the number of persons that the public would want to dispose of in this manner. Moreover, the public itself objects when these facilities become snake pits, as is very likely to happen in an over-crowded, understaffed institution, where there is little hope for release. One might add that it is inhumane—besides being illegal —to lock a mentally ill person in a cell for an indeterminate sentence because he pilfers groceries or frightens children.

On the other hand, if the administrator adheres rigidly to his therapeutic philosophy for patients, he can be viewed as, and in fact is, callous to the genuine concerns of the community. The fact that the number of crimes committed by mental patients is probably no greater, and may even be less, than those committed by the "normal" population is of little interest to the community. An attempted rape by a presumably hospitalized person who had committed such an act before has an undeniably greater signifi-cance to the public than a similar act committed by someone whose prior behavior has not brought him into the hands of public agencies.

The public rightly asks, as they asked us, "Is there no way to weed out the dangerous or the obnoxious and protect us from them? Why can't those patients be locked up?" The actuality is that there is no simple way to make this distinction. For example, at our community meeting, many members insisted that all court cases be sent to a maximum security hospital. It was difficult for them to believe that the majority of court cases are *not* dangerous, consisting as they do mostly of harmless alcoholics. By contrast, more than a few who come from routes other than the court *are* potentially violent. There is no clear-cut rule of thumb that would readily divide the patients into categories that could be easily explained to the public.

In short, the administrator must pursue his open-door policy as a general principle, even though this means being out of tune with large segments of the public. When the issue is in doubt he must support the patient, rather than the public. In practice, this commitment is always tempered by the demands of reality. The administrator can never be so emotionally removed from the public's point of view as to create a backlash that could pre-cipitously wipe out many gains, for example, by the community insisting that armed guards patrol the hospital grounds or that sentinels be placed at all exits.

Moreover, his responsibility to the public is very great. He must seriously consider every possible measure that would increase their sense of security, while not unduly and illegitimately restrict-ing the freedom of the patients. Indeed, in many instances, these two goals are complementary rather than mutually antagonistic. For example, at the community meeting, we could agree with the citizens that ward personnel had tended to relax the screening of patients suitable for ground privileges. Administration pointed out that it is as harmful to the patient as it is to the public to let a badly confused person wander around at will in the community without supervision or to expose a poorly controlled individual to the provocations of freedom. True, some of these patients might escape anyway, but the hospital has the clear responsibility not to invite such escapes by an indifferent attitude.

The community representatives rightly challenged us to make a more exact diagnosis of the potential risk to the community of each patient that enters the hospital. The hospital is, of course, concerned about anyone who is physically dangerous to himself or to others. But, as is clear from the complaints made at the meeting, there is a wide range of behavior that is threatening or obnoxious to the public, short of physical violence.

For the clearly dangerous, intensive study should be made to determine whether maximum-security sections should be established in every state hospital. This kind of setup has its difficulties. A ward for so-called dangerous patients can easily serve as a temptation for some staff to transfer to this section anyone who does not meet their standards or who provokes them. In addition, the very label *dangerous* is likely to heighten a patient's perception of himself as a menace and to bring his behavior more into line with this image rather than to work against it. No program for separate care for dangerous patients should be undertaken unless it provides an adequately trained staff, an active rehabilitation program to reclaim lives rather than merely to segregate them, and a research team to investigate the causes and treatment of antisocial behavior.

The administrator could then agree with some of the suggestions of the community representatives. But it cannot be glossed over that extremely severe problems remain regarding the handling of disruptive and obnoxious behavior. Every day an open hospital admits patients who are not only a potential menace to the community, but also to the hospital ward staff, which is comprised largely of women, and not of tough guards. For example, a man who has just savagely beaten his wife is admitted in a highly agitated state. If he is very disturbed and very menacing, he may well be secluded until he can be sufficiently treated so that he is no longer a threat to others. But suppose he is only *somewhat* disturbed and only *somewhat* menacing. In such an instance, the admitting physician may decide that he is not likely to beat up anybody and that he should not be secluded. His wife and female attendants, however, may have a different view of the matter and not wish to expose themselves to that "not likely" chance, which threatens them more directly than it does the person making the decision. They may argue very strongly not only for seclusion, but even, in many instances, for transfer to a maximum-security institution. What the decision ultimately is in such cloudy instances depends very much upon the attitude of the top administrator which filters down to all levels of staff.

Such extremely problematic instances could be multiplied ad infinitum: the man who goes home for a visit and occasionally abuses his children verbally in a frightening and noxious manner; the day patient who occasionally drives dangerously; the woman who occasionally exhibits herself when permitted to be in the community. The superintendent and hospital staff are constantly balancing incompletely understood gains and costs of different policies. What is the harm to the patient of being locked up or deprived of town privileges compared to the risks to the community if he is given more freedom? Our community representatives asked us to decide these highly complex issues always in *their* favor and when in doubt to restrict the patient. This was something we could not do. And it would do little good to remind them at the height of the controversy that they would not like to see themselves or their relatives handled in this fashion if they had the misfortune to be hospitalized.

One thing the administrator can do is to convert the kind of crisis confrontation we had with the community after the rape incident into a more continuing and less heated dialogue and process of mutual education. It is a fact that citizens who are likely to become most aroused after such an occurrence will include many who are not in accord with a progressive philosophy. But the very act of coming into the institution to discuss the issue with the administration reveals energy and concern. At least some of these people could with guidance become more sympathetic to the dilemmas and varied responsibilities of hospital staff. Moreover, without such counsel, some could become really destructive agitators against the community approach to the treatment of mental illness. Too often, we tend to regard such incidents as crises to be survived, rather than as opportunities to be explored. We breathe a sigh of relief when it looks as though the community has calmed down enough to leave quietly, perhaps temporarily appeased by what are really only very partial solutions to the problems of a state hospital in an urban area. It may bring temporary peace, but it is really not enough for the hospital, the community, and the legislators to agree that they will make every effort to get additional security personnel. Perhaps more important than anything else would be a sustained process of mutual talking together, mutual suggestions as to ways of dealing with problems. It should not take a crisis to bring together representatives of the hospital and the community to discuss issues of treatment—such as the open-door policy—that have direct and problematic consequences for the immediate community.

This issue is not limited to the state mental hospital. It confronts every community mental health center, every rehabilitation center, every aftercare facility. We know, for example, of several halfway houses that had to be temporarily closed because neighborhood people became upset about the real or alleged misbehavior of former hospitalized patients who were living there. The patients were not violent, but they did sometimes behave in a manner that many community people found hard to tolerate. Certain particularly hostile citizens were able to invoke previously overlooked zoning regulations and were successful in closing down these highly worthy efforts. We also know of a very successful summer camp for patients that could only come into being after long and arduous meetings with the community at which the patients' possible disruptive behavior was thoroughly discussed. (The camp organizers made sure that prominent community persons sympathetic to the project were present to counteract opinion against the plan and to help sway the undecided vote in favor of having the summer facility.)

We need to learn a good deal more about how to deal with the community's concern—which arguments more effectively mobilize their interest and which more effectively lessen their fears. We also have to know what kinds of persons are best suited to be spokesmen for these arguments and what kinds of discussion settings most enhance their effectiveness.

A full consideration of the issues of the community's tolerance of the mentally ill would lead us far afield. Here it is sufficient to underscore once again the importance of the administrator's not yielding too readily to the pressures stemming from lack of tolerance. The capacity to withstand opposition, not only to an open-door policy but also to other aspects of his treatment program, is an important prerequisite of any administrator. This is particularly the case when the leader is trying to introduce innovative programs on multiple fronts. There will always be many inside and outside the hospital who will complain bitterly about some aspect of his plan. Pursuing an eclectic philosophy, he cannot even count on a consistent lineup of support and opposition. Friends who back him when he launches a research effort may be opposed when he pursues a community program and vice versa. Not only is his toughness constantly tested, but also his political sense, using the word not pejoratively, but with its best meaning. It will do him little good to pride himself on his uncompromising idealism if he lacks the internal and external support to implement his ideas. But he will also fail if he is not prepared to face heated opposition and demands that he slow down, that he limit patients' freedom, that he abandon this or that program, or that he otherwise deviate from the course he has charted for the hospital.

REFERENCE

1. Joint Commission on Mental Illness and Health, *Action for Mental Health,* final report of the Commission (New York: Basic Books, 1961).

CHAPTER 4

Decentralization Through Unitization

As we noted in the prologue, the needs and demands of an ever-increasing population have been accompanied by a kind of giant-ism in all our public institutions. One proposed solution to some of the problems of these elephantine, depersonalized establish-ments is decentralization. Although decentralization means differ-ent things to different people, in the context of the state mental hospital, decentralization, or unitization as it is commonly called, involves breaking up the institution into semiautonomous units, each with its own admission service, treatment programs for both acute and chronic patients, and transitional and aftercare programs. Each unit has the responsibility for serving a specific part of the community; in effect, it is a small community mental health center, with its own geographic base. Even the reader who is unfamiliar with the many new developments in community mental health will recognize the similiarity between this approach and recent trends in education.

Decentralization formalizes or makes highly explicit a principle we tried to follow even before unitization was considered at Bos-ton State; namely, the delegation of responsibility and maximum participation in decision-making. Unitization embodied this con-cept by having semiautonomous divisions within the hospital, each led by a unit director, and each having considerable oppor-tunity to devise its own ways of coping with its own problems. Whatever arguments the members of a given unit might have about authority, responsibility, or decision-making, they would have considerable freedom to work it out among themselves.

The principle of unitization accorded well with our multiple-treatment ideology. If the different unit directors had different kinds of psychiatric orientations, then each could have the freedom to develop his own particular style or philosophy to the maximum under a system that gave great latitude to unit autonomy. In a sense, this plan has important similiarities to the philosophic underpinnings of our state-federal system, which was in part designed to allow for considerable experimentation by the individual states. Innovations could be tested, with the damage of negative ones being limited in its effect and with the example of positive changes being available for others to emulate.

A third attractive feature of unitization was that it was in harmony with the developing regional plans for the state. Instead of a gargantuan hospital serving a gargantuan community, smaller, decentralized hospitals could serve smaller and more accessible community catchment areas. Community psychiatry is difficult enough to accomplish and, in its true sense, remains to be accomplished. But it surely never will be achieved unless the ground is laid for person-to-person contact between the hospital and the community. At Boston State, it was simply out of the question for staff of a service with a heterogeneous array of patients from every part of greater Boston to get to know, for example, the small social agencies of twenty or so different communities. Indeed, the hospital's chronic complaint that it was understaffed had to do in part with the inefficient organization of the staff's tasks. Even if there had been many more workers, the prodigious job of getting to know a city-wide community would have made them give up even before they started. The situation vis-à-vis the community is reminiscent of the story told by a psychiatrist that he had never had so much free time as when he had to take care of five hundred patients all by himself: it was so difficult to do anything that he did nothing.

A final attractive feature of decentralization was that it helped ameliorate the distinction between "good" (acute) patients and "bad" (chronic) ones. The common practice among small centers has been to select "good," young acute patients for treatment and send "bad" ones to the large state hospital. But at Boston State, we were further educated that such distinctions are not easily discarded. Even in a state hospital, there was the "good" place, for "good" patients—the reception building, which processed about twenty-four hundred patients a year. All those accepted for inpatient care were first hospitalized in this building of about one hundred and eighty beds. By virtue of its function, this admission area had a high concentration of staff, training programs, and professional activities. If, after three months, the patients in reception did not make the grade of discharge or show real promise of doing so, they were transferred to long-term treatment centers, which were more honestly described at the hospital as chronic wards.

As one result of this procedure, fifteen hundred patients had accumulated over the years in long-stay buildings, where the staff-patient ratio was far less favorable, professional activities and training programs were almost negligible, and the pace of therapeutic work was slowed to a walk. An occasional exception was the "interesting" patient whom the psychiatrist-resident had chosen for psychoanalytically oriented psychotherapy.

A cardinal aspect of unitization, then, was that it would ameliorate, and perhaps eliminate this distinction between acute and chronic patients, at least in a service sense. That is, each unit was to be responsible for all patients from its catchment area, and transfers were disallowed. Obviously, decentralization in and of itself does not necessarily preclude staff's giving more attention to acute, responsive patients and less attention to chronic, apathetic ones. But it does mean that each unit has to be constantly confronted with its failures rather than shifting them off to some remote part of the hospital, where the very label of "chronic service" helps ingrain the chronic features of the transferred patient.

The Process: Early Phases

The administrator did not come to Boston State with any specific idea of decentralizing the institution although, as we have mentioned, the goals of unitization were syntonic with his overall philosophy of administration. However, a few key staff members spoke about it very enthusiastically. Their fervor, plus independent study of the literature, made him increasingly receptive to the notion of implementing some form of decentralization.

Initially, when the subject came up for serious discussion in 1965, its problematic features received far more attention than its advantages. Many staff members complained that there were insufficient personnel to man separate units on each service; there was need for more centralized departments than unitization allowed in order to provide for staff training and recruitment; chronic patients had to be handled differently from acute patients and hence the two groups could not be housed together, and so on.

It soon appeared that unitization might very well represent an upheaval of tremendous magnitude to the hospital. The administrator saw his task during the early phases of this development as furthering the exploration of the possibilities of unitization, but at the same time recognizing the objections, rational or irrational, to the plan. He tried to communicate to opponents of decentralization that its merits could not be summarily dismissed by saying "we can't" and to advocates that its implementation required both a clearer plan than had yet been presented and a wider staff agreement in favor of the idea.

An early step was the report of the three men who had visited several unitized hospitals (chapter 1). They claimed that they had "seen the future and it works." Staff response to their enthusiasm could be broken down into three categories: those who did not care a whit one way or the other, those who said decentralization had no major advantages and should not be attempted, and those who saw substantial gains and wanted it tried sooner or later.

Administration was sufficiently encouraged by the report of the three men to request that they formulate a definite design for decentralization, although the decision about actual implementation, if and particularly when, had not yet been settled. To fulfill this request, the proponents would be compelled to be

more specific about actual details of the operation so the opponents would have something concrete to which they could
respond. In a relatively short time, the unitization committee
offered a plan that in its major outline looked something like
the following.

The decentralized hospital would consist of four basic units,
each serving a section of the community. We were governed
in this decision by the prevailing notion derived from federal
guidelines that a comprehensive community mental health center
should serve a population of not less than seventy-five thousand
and not more than two hundred thousand. Since Boston State
served about eight hundred thousand people, the division came
close to the maximum figure. The choice for fewer units rather
than more had a practical basis. Each unit had to include leadership individuals representing psychiatry, psychology, social work,
nursing, rehabilitation, and occupational therapy. Leaders with
a potential for developing dynamic units who could simultaneously attract and hold the best possible staff, teach students of all
disciplines, and pursue innovations in patient care were indeed
exceedingly rare. Even with four units, we were stretching our
resources perilously thin. Also, according to the plan, the geriatric
unit, which consisted of patients older than sixty, coming from
all sections of the city, was to remain unaffected, as was the
medical-surgical unit, for obvious reasons.

It was also planned that at or about the time of unitization, a
number of acute patients would be transferred from the reception
building (the acute-care unit) to the various long-term treatment
centers, and a certain number of chronic patients would be transferred to the reception building. With this immediate exchange,
the "chronic" buildings would now have sufficient recovery flow
to insure bed space to handle their geographically designated
new admissions. Moreover, since two long-term service areas consisted entirely of women and one entirely of men, it was also
planned that there would be some exchange of patients to provide a mixed-sex distribution on each service. Thus, our earlier
goal of integration of sexes was accelerated by the unitization plan.

It can be readily seen that the actual spelling-out of the unitization plan could be very provocative to those who had been opposed to or skeptical about the idea. An extremely radical reorganization of the hospital was involved, with a D-day, or perhaps better a U-day, that would entail shifting around some patients from every service. Not only would there be changes in function, but there would also be changes in human relationships. We frequently speak of how patients become attached to certain places and people, but neglect to mention that staff members also become attached to patients—for right and wrong reasons.

In any event, a storm of controversy now erupted, particularly when a date several months hence was proposed by the unitization committee as the probable time for the change. Just as the plan had become more sharply formulated, so had the opposing arguments become more precise. The administrator encouraged the give and take of ideas by making the subject of unitization a prime topic at the various hospital meetings he chaired and urged others to do the same. The objections he met and the counterarguments he offered are discussed below.

Staff Shortage

The first objection, and the one that was to remain the most serious throughout the period of decision, concerned the alleged shortage of staff to fulfill the demands of decentralization. In order to understand this objection, we shall detail some background information.

The allocation design in effect at Boston State prior to unitization (and the traditional one in most state hosiptals) involved, as we mentioned earlier, the concentration of all acute cases in one building, which had a much higher staff-patient ratio than the rest of the hospital. This density of staff was justified partly on the grounds that most acute patients responded swiftly to treatment and hence should be given top priority to help facilitate their return to the community. Also, and perhaps more important from staff's point of view, it was justified on the grounds that acute patients are much more apt to act in antisocial, disruptive ways than the more predictable, apathetic, inactive chronic ones. Thus, the volatile atmosphere of the reception building demanded a huge preponderance of scarce male attendants who could come quickly to one another's aid during emergencies.

Now, the hospital "radicals," aided and abetted by the administrator, were proposing that the previously consolidated unpredictable patients be distributed throughout the hospital. Where were the additional staff coming from to man acute admissions on *four* services?

This question could partly be answered by saying that the present chronic services would get some additional help from the reception building once that unit was no longer required to take in all the new admissions. Although this partial answer provided some comfort to staff members in the long-term buildings, it was met with considerable objection by those in the acute unit. They considered themselves the elite of the hospital; being sent to another unit would reduce their prestige. Moreover, they would lose skilled personnel in return for a group of chronic patients they were not trained to handle.

The administrator pointed out that they would experience a real gain through the reduction of their admission load. For one relatively small building to carry the full load of alcoholics, drug addicts, and excited, belligerent, violent, and threatening patients resulted in a frenetic pace of activities that was as unhealthy in its own way as the torpor of the long-term treatment building. Indeed, because of its rising admission rate, the reception building had long since passed its peak of efficiency and seemed to be going downhill in terms of morale and patient care. Therefore, relief from the great burden of acute patients seemed mandatory.

We may add, parenthetically, that one administrative technique used to stimulate the reception building's desire for unitization was to partially close the valve governing transfers between the acute and chronic services. By order, staff had to get specific administrative permission before they could transfer a case. With a rising admission rate, and now with less freedom to relocate patients, the acute service became more receptive to the decentralization plan, which would diffuse the pressure of admissions over three other services.

A further answer to the issue of staff shortage was that several hospitals had in fact unitized with considerably less staff than at Boston State and without the catastrophic consequences predicted by the opponents of decentralization. It was also felt that the very experience of dealing with more responsive patients would give a psychological lift to the long-term treatment services and that the reality of acute cases would, in many ways, be less frightening than the fantasies about them.

Reorganization of Professional Departments

Once again, some background information is necessary for the reader to understand the full implication for this concern about the fate of professional departments under unitization.

Prior to unitization, a given professional functioned within the traditional system under a setup of "multiple subordinancy," to use Jules Henry's term.[1] For example, a psychologist reported not only to the chief of the service to which he was assigned but also to the director of psychology. A psychiatric resident reported not only to a senior service psychiatrist but also to the director of psychiatric training. This system had the advantage of protecting the trainee to some degree from inordinate service demands that interfered with his learning. The chief of his professional department could negotiate with the service chief in disputed areas over the relative importance of service versus education.

Unitization was seen as a threat to the power of the professional departments. For a small department, it represented a dislocation in a purely geographical sense, as well as in other aspects. For example, the psychologists had always been located in the reception building, where their main clinical work consisted in testing new patients and learning psychotherapy with a few selected acute patients—all under the fairly close direction of the chief psychologist. Under unitization, these few psychologists would be distributed among the four units, where their tasks might vary greatly, depending on the needs of the unit, and the negotiations between the unit chief and the psychologist assigned to that unit. True, nothing prevented the psychologists from reassembling in one place for courses in supervision under the guidance of the director of psychology. But no one could gainsay that unitization represented a major shift in the functioning of that service.

A somewhat different threat was posed to a very large department, such as nursing. Here, the director of nurses was concerned not only about education but also about the weakening of his power to disperse his staff as he saw fit. In a traditional system, he could move them around from building to building in the face of particular emergencies or specific shortages; in the unit system, he feared he would lose this flexibility and power.

Although it was contemplated that under unitization department heads would function more in terms of recruitment, training, consultation, and research, rather than in terms of supervision and immediate direction of clinical work, these department heads feared—not without reason—that recruitment particularly might eventually pass out of their hands. There was already a tendency at the hospital for smaller specialized units, such as the adolescent and drug addiction services, to recruit their own personnel. The nursing director, for example, was understandably anxious: without a strong centralized department, a highly aggressive unit director might be able to fill empty positions more readily than other directors, to the neglect of the needs of the hospital as a whole.

The administrator was not particularly impressed by the argument against decentralization on the grounds that it would weaken the professional departments. Indeed, his predilection for flexible role-functioning was much more consonant with the idea of unit teams than it was with the whole concept of strict professional identities of nurse, psychiatrist, or social worker, reinforced by powerful department heads. The very model of highly specialized departments reflected the medical approach to the treatment of psychiatric problems in which it was conceived that the mentally ill could be divided up into parts the way the physically ill are, with a particular specialist responsible for a particular section of the patient's body or a particular aspect of his total care.

However, the recent history of psychiatric treatment has suggested that what the mental patient needs most is a continuous, unbroken relationship with one person. Just as he finds bewildering and upsetting a rapid shift from place to place with its disruptions in human relationships, he also finds perplexing a shift from one person to another for various specialized treatments. More and more, the aim was for one person to have overall responsibility for a given patient, even though he would make use of a wide range of consultants: rehabilitation, social work, and so on. Obviously, this key person could not be confined to the ranks of a few high-level professional disciplines, if for no other reason than the shortage of such people. All personnel would have to be seen as potentially capable of fulfilling this role.

In short, the thrust in treatment was toward the clinical "generalist" who could perform a wide variety of functions with patients and know where to turn for consultative help when that was necessary. The administrator preferred to make this kind of flexibility the basis of functioning from which, later, more specialized roles might develop rather than attempt to move toward flexibility from prearranged, more rigid professional demarcations. The unit plan was fully consonant with this overall philosophy.

Although the substantive arguments based on the weakening of professional departments could be challenged, the *personal* feelings of professional chiefs demanded very serious consideration. They would have to function quite differently when their subordinates became attached to semiautonomous units and unit chiefs who would gain their primary loyalty. The anxiety of the department heads was heightened by reports that at one hospital, the positions of chiefs of professional departments had disappeared as a result of decentralization. No one likes to have his job shot out from under him. It is an obvious but frequently overlooked point that in any redefinition of a job, the future role should be made as clear and as palatable as possible for the one who must give up established tasks and assume new ones.

In the case of professional chiefs, the administrator emphasized that with unitization the more important functions of teaching, consultation, and research would not only remain in their hands, but would gain even greater prominence than with the present system. If the department heads identified strongly with these functions, the change toward unitization did not appear so personally disruptive; if they were more concerned with the purely administrative aspects of their position, the reorganization was very disturbing.

Catchment Areas

Some persons favored the idea of unitization insofar as it provided continuity of care for the patient; that is, they liked the idea of the patient "belonging" to one unit. However, they objected to each unit being linked with a specific geographic area for several reasons.

First, they felt that such a division would lead to a new kind of segregation of patients, now not on the basis of acute versus chronic, but on the basis of the racial or social class composition of the particular community area the unit served. (Racial imbalance was already an explosive issue at that time in the school system of Boston, which was being confronted with de facto segregation in the classroom.) They also felt that through the idiosyncrasies of one or another catchment area, certain kinds of patient pathology might pile up in one or another unit. For example, the unit whose catchment area included the skid-row district might be overwhelmed with alcoholics; the unit serving a roominghouse area might be top-heavy with lonely, depressed people.

Second, they felt that the rationale for the elaborate process of linking units with community divisions was weak. The linkage was *supposed* to provide closer contact and relationships between the hospital and the community, but the reality of staff shortage would make a chimera of the idea of the hospital getting into the community.

On the basis of both these reasons, they argued for a *random* rotation of new admissions in terms of patient composition. In addition, a random rotation would insure an accurate and steady patient load for each unit, whereas under the catchment principle, there might be a flood of admissions into one unit on a given week and very few on another.

These objections were forceful ones and had to be taken seriously. Indeed, the first argument concerning a proper social, racial, and economic balance of patients on each unit influenced our design in relating units to catchment areas. We tried to arrange it so that each geographic division would achieve this desired composition. Thus, one unit that initially was to receive patients only from middle-class sections of the city had its community responsibility enlarged to include a substantial underprivileged area. However, only time would tell how successful we were in preventing ghettoization or other forms of segregated groupings of patients within the hospital. We also allowed for periodic reexamination of our community divisions in case such patient balance was not achieved or in case some community divisions were providing more admissions into their respective units and others less than had been originally planned.

The second objection—that the units would be too thinly staffed to involve themselves with the community—was more basic but had less validity. If a state mental hospital were to wait for sufficient staff it would *never* make any innovations. True, it was hard to conceive how a small band of unit professionals could engage in, say, consultation to the schools in its catchment area and at the same time handle their load of patient-oriented problems. Still, it was hoped that the unit-community linkage would accomplish at least two important things.

First, it would facilitate a closer cooperation between the unit and the various health and welfare agencies in the community to which the unit was attached. It should be noted that the unitization plan called for several units to be backup areas for small, university-based mental health centers, which had their own catchment areas to serve. Decentralization facilitated the collaboration between these inpatient units at Boston State and the outpatient and consultation services at the mental health centers.

Second, as we have suggested earlier, it would help the hospital staff develop an overall community orientation. Undoubtedly, this would have to proceed slowly. But over time, we hoped—and we may add parenthetically that our hope was partially borne out—that the inpatient staff members would see the value of closer community collaboration more clearly when they had a circumscribed area to cover. They would, for example, come to realize that to spare one capable nurse to devote herself to working with other community agencies on the follow-up care of discharged patients might, in the long run, significantly reduce the readmission rate. This kind of staff allocation was in fact what happened on one of the most inpatient-oriented units in the hospital, an allocation which we believe would never have occurred without unitization.

It is worth underscoring that it is important for the administrator not to permit current obstacles to stop movements into the future which, in the long run, will ameliorate the very shortages that presumably prevent the innovation. The administrator, of course, cannot be so unrealistic as to dream wildly—or even worse, act too precipitously—concerning new developments. Indeed, a few of our community-oriented people sharply alienated more traditionally minded staff members by presenting plans for working in the community as though they could and should be adopted overnight. But granted the pressures of reality, the administrator must still do everything to support whatever seems to have a chance, as decentralization did, of providing a basis for further growth and improvement.

Education

We have already mentioned that the professional chiefs feared that unitization might lessen their hold, including their educational impact, on staff members and students from their special disciplines. A further objection along educational lines had to do with the particular implications of unitization for service assignments.

Prior to unitization, psychiatric residents, for example, were assigned to specific services for three or four months of rotation. This changing of services permitted them to learn about different kinds of patients and exposed them to the different styles and philosophies of various service chiefs. A grave disadvantage of this arrangement was that it meant the constant breaking of ties between the student and service mentors, colleagues, and patients. It sharply violated the service principle of continuity of treatment in the name of the educational principle of diversity of instruction. The proponents of unitization argued that decentralization would provide a heterogeneity of patients on *each* unit and thus greatly reduce the need for the student to rotate from service to service. It was envisioned that a resident might spend his entire first year on one basic unit and get more specialized kinds of experience, for example, with geriatric or home treatment patients, in his second or third year.

The educational argument against this by some was that if continuity of treatment were respected, the residents would be exposed to only one service tutor, at least in their first year. According to their predilections, some senior staff members thought it would be a disaster for a resident to have only Dr. X as his chief, whereas others thought it would be a grave misfortune if he had only Dr. Y.

Although this concern had merit, it stimulated thought about the teaching mix that would be available on each unit, a subject to be discussed in more detail in the chapter on training. Suffice it here to say also that the administrator never did insist on an absolute rule on length of service assignments. He hoped wherever possible to maximize continuity of treatment as long as it did not do great injustice to the educational needs of the student.

The Process: Later Phases

Over time, in the give-and-take of arguments about unitization, staff's earlier positions became somewhat realigned. Far fewer were now indifferent to the whole issue. Although many were still opposed, they were aware, and accurately so, that decentralization in some form or another was going to take place.

The main debate now shifted from the question of *whether* to the question of *how.* The most important consideration now was: should decentralization begin with only one unit or should it encompass the entire hospital right from the start?

Once again, there were three positions. Members of one proposed unit, which was destined to be the community mental health center for the major part of the hospital's own immediate catchment area, had already made considerable, and tenacious, efforts toward providing comprehensive programs. Through a variety of imaginative aftercare programs, such as foster-home placement and rehabilitative day care, among others, they had greatly reduced their census of long-term patients. Moreover, even during the discussion about unitization, they had begun experimenting successfully in admitting directly to their unit certain acute patients from their proposed catchment area. Because of their enterprise, they had received a somewhat disproportionate share of the hospital's resources to further their innovations. The idea of total hospital decentralization threatened them because they feared this help might be withdrawn in order to meet the unitization needs of the other services. Their argument was that if they were further assisted in their present direction, they could continue to experiment and thus show the rest of the hospital the proper way to build a comprehensive unit serving a catchment area.

They also presented in great detail the problems requiring solution before decentralization—problems so vast in scope that, in their opinion, step-by-step unitization, one unit at a time, was practically mandatory. These problems included definition of the catchment area; organization of the community for acceptance and participation in unitization; continuity of patient care from admission through to community placement; renovation and repair of physical plants; establishment of an adequate record system; installation of a proper telephone and call system; role definition and consequent realignment of loyalties of professionals; and complexities introduced by training demands.

The second position, one at the other extreme, was that the opportunity to decentralize should be seized in order to make every service a truly comprehensive unit. Granted certain unavoidable exceptions, such as the ailing in the medical-surgical building, all patients, even geriatric ones in good physical condition, should belong with the unit serving their area. Various special services, such as home treatment, the outpatient clinic, and the adolescent unit, should also be decentralized. That is, they should be broken up and staff from these groupings assigned to every unit so that each could have its own personnel for home visits, outpatient treatment, and so on. In a sense, this was following the logic of unitization to its ultimate conclusion; *all* services for patients from a given catchment area should be integratively coordinated under one roof.

The third position, which represented a compromise between the two preceding ones, acquired precise form through the process of discussion and argument that occurred during the hectic months just prior to actual unitization. The idea of proceeding with only one unit was rejected on several grounds. Although it had been useful to have some pilot efforts in the unit direction, to continue building up one area to the neglect of the others was to add an unbearable sense of friction between this privileged unit and the rest of the hospital. Indeed, so distasteful was this idea even to many opponents of unitization that they rallied to the cause of an enlarged decentralization if only to avoid the further gaining of privileges by the model unit. In a certain real sense, the hospital could not long survive half-unitized and half-centralized, particularly where basic inpatient services were involved. Moreover, the more entrenched one unit became with its own plans and development, the harder it would be for that unit eventually to undergo the inevitable dislocations stemming from a larger decentralization. Indeed, some of the results of such an entrenchment were already evident in the furor raised by the privileged unit over the issue of hospital-wide unitization.

The second position was also untenable. Although a relatively *total* decentralization was the ultimate goal, its immediate implementation would be disastrous. Some of our specialized services were conceived as innovative, experimental efforts, and their high morale depended crucially on their being able to function as semiautonomous units. Were their relatively small staff to be dispersed through a mechanical division among the four units, they would lose the pioneering spirit and zeal that characterized their functioning.

This latter issue was connected with another problematic point. There was undoubtedly an egalitarian thrust to decentralization and some of its ardent supporters wanted to see this particular aspect rigidly adhered to. Units would have staff assigned to them strictly on the basis of the number of patients expected from their catchment area, and practically all employees would be lumped together in a personnel reservoir from which the subsequent divisions would be made. Without question, this process of personnel division could become a battleground for unit chiefs and staff, as shown by the animus already expressed toward the unit and toward certain new services, which were seen by many as privileged in their staffing patterns.

The compromise position, and the one the administrator supported, was as follows. The one model unit would not be maintained, but, as originally planned, there would be four units, to serve all patients younger than sixty. At the same time, special innovative units would be permitted to continue in their present mode of functioning. This did not prevent their helping the four basic units develop their own special programs, but it did preserve the integrity of the demonstration efforts. Moreover, an absolute equality in staffing patterns would not be applied. Such a division would be detrimental to certain special programs and teaching strengths some services had already developed. To divide at one fell swoop all these resources equally around the hospital could have deleterious consequences. Thus, the foster-home program, which had been developed largely by nurses on one particular unit, was permitted to continue in force on that unit after decentralization, although it was expected that the nurses would offer their specialized skills to other units. The reception building, which was particularly endowed with senior psychiatric personnel, still received, after unitization, a somewhat disproportionate share of residents in order to make use of the teaching skills available on that service.

Undoubtedly, this compromise position left many dissatisfied. However, in the administrator's view, it represented the best way of making a major step forward without unduly disrupting different facets of the hospital's operation.

By the time this plan was firmly decided on, in the early summer of 1966, many months of heated discussion had passed. Some persons who had been colleagues in arms for unitization parted company when the issue became one unit at a time versus four units all at once. Tempers were frayed. By now, people were eager to get moving, to end the controversies. They wanted a unitization date, as though only that kind of concreteness would make the whole enterprise real after so much discussion.

During the summer the administrator tried to achieve the fullest possible acceptance of the plan. However, since summer vacations have a way of diluting intense emotions and restoring perspective, he waited until after Labor Day to announce the exact details about unitization and to set the date for the move. He notified staff at the first large fall meeting that unitization was to take place sometime in October. He deliberately set the date close at hand in order to mitigate the consequences of further, prolonged anxiety. He also avoided setting a highly specific date so that staff could not express its hostility in a delay that constituted an express negation of the administrator's order. The more indeterminate date of "sometime in October" permitted the administrator the opportunity, which he indeed utilized, of waiting until the very last day of the month to implement the decision.

The Deed Is Done

As with many other changes at the hospital, the actual unitization was far less traumatic than had been predicted by many. Once the date was set, anxieties were rapidly converted into the energies demanded of logistics. Every echelon of the hospital rallied to mapping and executing the strategy of transferring patients, reallocating staff, making buildings and wards ready to accommodate their new charges, packing suitcases, and so on. It would be beyond the scope of this narrative to present a full picture of what U-day or its immediate aftermath was like. We shall limit ourselves to describing some highlights that have particular implications for effecting this kind of momentous change:

1. One of the most important aspects of unitization day in terms of patients was adequate preparation. Some staff, particularly those caring for chronic patients, thought too much discussion of the coming change would only upset and confuse their charges. Hence, they gave patients who were due to be transferred very little notice of what was to happen. On another chronic service, the whole issue of separation was discussed in far more detail. The patients in this service reacted initially with more grief during the changeover, but they made a better adjustment after they moved. The patients who were not so well prepared tended to wander around for some time after unitization, complaining because they were no longer in their familiar settings.

2. The unanticipated consequences of the change were sometimes far more problematic than the anticipated ones. For example, the stress acute patients would put on the long-term treatment services was expected. Indeed, after unitization, there remained much concern about proper staffing of the various admission units. But there was also a great deal of satisfaction on these services that they now at last were dealing with more responsive patients. What had been insufficiently predicted was the degree of strain that would be felt by staff of the former reception unit when it now had to care for transferred long-term patients. They were not afraid of these patients, but, initially, they were very discouraged by them.

3. The argument that unitization would require more staff was refuted by the experience. Shortages of staff were keenly felt, but the gains of unitization seemed to outweigh its disadvantages.

What Did Unitization Accomplish?

There is no doubt that unitization had precipitated the greatest upheaval that Boston State had had in years. However, the act of decentralization infused the institution with a more dynamic spirit, even while it was suffering from the strains of transition.

The unit system diminished the corrosive, sometimes inhumane, distinctions between acute and chronic patients by putting responsibility for both under one authority. In some areas, social mixing of acute and chronic patients helped further to submerge the difference. In any case, since staff could no longer transfer "bad" or "unresponsive" patients to some other service, all units had to face the continuing problem of developing more successful ways of dealing with long-term patients.

Responsibility for a geographic area enhanced interest in community resources and referral agencies, as well as family participation, aftercare, and preventive services. Since all of Boston had to be divided up into districts, and boundaries were left to us, we arranged our geographic areas in relation to hospitals that regularly transferred to us a major number of their chronically ill patients. We thus strengthened our clinical and teaching programs by closer collaboration with these centers.

Finally, and most important, unitization forced the development of more treatment teams, each responsible for and in contact with smaller groups of patients. New opportunities for leadership positions were opened up, not only to psychiatrists, but eventually to psychologists, social workers, and nurses. Thus, unitization challenged each unit administrator to develop the most flexible, comprehensive program of treatment, research, and training possible. Competition among units stimulated bolder thinking and action. In short, unitization released new kinds of creative therapeutic relationships, catalyzing ideas which had been latent for years, but which required such a major organizational change to emerge.

In Retrospect

The administrative pros and cons of a long period of uncertainty and discussion about an anticipated major reorganizational change are many. In our particular example of decentralization, more than a year of serious discussion had elapsed prior to the implementation of the decision.

There were certain disadvantages to this delay, and these will be discussed below. However, there is considerable wisdom in an administrator not getting caught up in the demands for a quick decision about a controversial issue. When changes of great moment are at stake, the process of clarifying difficulties and trying to resolve differences of opinion is an important one. Administration believed that unless the many objections could be seriously dealt with, decentralization might end up so attentuated as to emerge a token thing, not worth all the commotion. If, on the other hand, the plan in its full dimension were ordered by heavy-handed administrative fiat, it could be sabotaged at lower levels, with the resultant chaos injurious to both patients and staff.

However, as we have already suggested, the lengthy process of decentralization was very much influenced by the administrator's own initial uncertainty about the wisdom of unitization at Boston State and his continuing questions as to its feasibility. But this by no means makes it a poor example for a book on administrative practice. Administrators must often involve themselves and their staffs in serious investigation of a possible major change without initially being sure that such a change is wise. They must also sometimes start the machinery for implementing such an innovation while allowing themselves the latitude of changing their minds should unforeseen obstacles arise.

Granted the uncertainties about the wisdom, timing, and nature of the unitization decision, there were advantages in the lengthy process leading to implementation. For one thing, by permitting his ambivalence to be felt, the administrator encouraged the fullest expression of views pro and con, particularly among senior personnel. This in turn allowed him to gain considerable information on which to base his ultimate decision. If an administrator comes on very strong in favor of a given policy right from the start, the weight of his authority may silence objecting voices. He has to take some objections into account in order to improve his plan and he must at least discuss others in order to elicit as much cooperation as possible. He can do neither if the complaints are not expressed. For example, his own openness to all arguments insured that he heard—and, indeed, he heard more than he cared to—about the very real staff shortages that decentralization could exacerbate. In order to relieve his own anxieties, as well as staff's, he had to look very thoroughly into all the details of personnel problems that might ensue subsequent to unitization.

Another advantage was that, in the absence of the administrator's taking a strong position, others would feel moved to do so, both pro and con. Although we have argued earlier that it is above all the top leader's responsibility to chart firmly the direction of the hospital, there are also advantages of his sometimes encouraging others not only to play a very major role in organizational change but also to take responsibility for meeting objections to the new proposals. Staff members can gain a valuable learning experience in standing up to the fire of opposition without administration backing them to the hilt. They must convince on the basis of the merits of their arguments rather than on the basis of being able to say "the boss wants." Furthermore, it is easier for staff to voice their objections to a lieutenant seeking votes for his cause than it is for them to criticize an actively campaigning administrator.

On balance, we believe that once administration's convictions had hardened in favor of unitization, it would have been wiser to proceed more rapidly, even with some inward lingering doubts. By preserving options to the last possible moment, more staff controversy and anxiety were generated than was necessary.

A few last words about the whole issue of consensus in regard to decision-making. Even if the administrator is relatively certain where he wants to go, he must win the support of others if he is actually going to get there successfully. But, as in all such questions, there are no absolutes. The critical pragmatic issue is how *much* support one needs from *how many* others. Because the unitization change was so basic, the administrator wanted to get considerable support from many others, particularly senior staff members, before he finally backed a plan and set a date. Whatever the enthusiasts of group process may argue, wholehearted unanimity cannot always be obtained in a large organization. There are too many crisscrossing, competing pressures and interests, as well as irrational anxieties and resistances for there to be true agreement.

In a sense, the protracted discussions did achieve a consensus of a certain kind. In addition to working through real objections, there was also the lukewarm agreement given to the actual plan out of fear that if our form of decentralization did not occur, another, worse kind, might triumph. There was also the consensus of exhaustion. Some people preferred to go ahead with some plan, indeed *any* plan, rather than have to endure any further talk. This kind of consensus, in fact, is not unique to our experience with unitization, but occurs often when there is protracted discussion about any decision.

In the absence of a genuine consensus and in the face of the kind of controversy that usually accompanies major change, somebody, at some point, has to make a decision that others will not like. One of the biggest theoretical and practical issues confronting all of us working in the human sector is the whole question of what is meant by group participation in decision-making. In the example of unitization of a large hospital, it is wise for the administrator or his deputy to obtain a full picture from *all* levels of staff as to their initial feelings about decentralization. This quest for opinion should be frankly stated as a search for advice and information, with the ultimate power of decision based not on a vote, but on the discretion of management. It is true that staff may be angered at such discussion if they believe that the administrator has already made up his mind and is just seeking to manipulate their consent for his choice. If he has not made up his mind, as the administrator had not in the early stages of unitization, there is no remedy for this complaint, except the frank statement of how things actually stand in the decision-making process. Once the choice is made, every effort should be expended at involving wide representation in working out the details of that decision.

REFERENCE

1. "Types of Institutional Structure," in *The Patient and the Mental Hospital,* ed. M. Greenblatt, D. J. Levinson, and R. H. Williams (Glencoe: Free Press, 1957), pp. 73–90.

PART II

Special Services

CHAPTER 5

The Adolescent
Consultation Service

In the context of this section, special projects are services that cut across unit lines to treat special kinds of patients, such as adolescents, drug addicts, and foster-home placements. Many of these projects embody a demonstration effort directed toward a particular goal and thus require a somewhat autonomous organizational structure. They often represent the pioneering, innovative edge of the hospital, from which concepts and practices can flow to be disseminated later, if proved successful, throughout the entire institution. However, the development and maintenance of special projects, especially in a hospital that is freeing itself from such delimiting distinctions as acute versus chronic services is highly problematic. It is also problematic in the ethos of a hospital that, aside from the distinction of acute versus chronic, is striving to maintain an equality in the distribution of resources, especially in terms of allotment of staff and other privileges.

In this chapter, using the adolescent consultation service as our example, we shall analyze many dilemmas arising in connection with such special units. We shall describe how the adolescent service came about and something of its functioning. However, our main focus will be on the administrative concepts and techniques in starting and nurturing such a service.

Adolescents in a State Hospital

Like many mental hospitals in the 1960s, Boston State was admitting even more young people than was warranted by the proportionally large adolescent population, as anticipated from the baby boom after World War II. This phenomenon was attributed to a specific increase among the young in emotional deviations, psychopathic behavior, and drug addiction. Everything was being blamed—affluence, poverty, family disorganization, too much sexual sophistication, sexual suppression, not enough sexual education, the pill, tensions and anxieties of the nuclear age, lack of religious education, and the stresses of urban living.

But regardless of the reason, the problem was vast, the need was pressing, and response had to be quick. The challenge to make a contribution to the better understanding and treatment of these sick adolescents was reinforced by a directive from the Massachusetts Department of Mental Health in February 1964 stating that "of major concern to the Department is the colossal growth of the population 15–24 years of age. In the four-year period (1958–1962), the number of new patients admitted at age 15–25 rose 35% for Massachusetts State hospitals."

Our most immediate response was to make a thorough survey of Boston State's adolescent population. We hoped that with this information, we could have a firm base on which to lay a plan for reasonable action. We asked a social worker with both clinical and research experience in the field of adolescence to conduct the study.[1] It is worthwhile to pause here to note that there was a serious shortage of social workers in the hospital. The chief of that department was strongly opposed, and with justification, to an experienced caseworker doing research rather than giving much needed service. Nevertheless, the administrator believed the need to be great enough to override the department head's objections and urged the social worker to continue as planned.

The interviewing and data-gathering encompassed the reception building, the chronic wards, and the outpatient facilities. The report was indeed sobering. We learned that more than 100 adolescents were admitted to the hospital per year; about 150 were in residence at some time during a given year, with another 60 being treated in outpatient facilities. A great majority had not gone beyond the first or second year of high school, had not acquired any job skills, and had not had any vocational training. About seventy percent had been away from ordinary community living and normal adolescent activities for some time; they had come from the courts, detention homes, mental hospitals, and schools for the retarded. Some were vagrants, homeless, and nomadic. Seventy-five percent of those admitted in 1963, for example, were released at least once during the year, but at the year's end most were again institutionalized, either at Boston State or elsewhere.

Prior to unitization, newly admitted adolescent patients were all housed in one facility—the reception building—spending their days and nights with alcoholics, acutely disturbed and often wildly psychotic men and women, as well as offenders sent to the hospital by the courts for observation. As with adult patients, those who showed no sign of improvement were sent to chronic buildings, although efforts were frequently made by interested staff members to keep them in the acute-care facility. But wherever they were, there was little for them to do. Some attended school classes on the hospital grounds, staffed by two teachers; others tried their hand at some form of occupational therapy. But by and large, their time was unstructured and their days purposeless. Most of them, though, did have a therapist—either a psychiatrist, a nurse, or a psychologist—and belonged to a therapy group. Psychopharmaceuticals were used sparingly. In some instances, formal conferences were held with parents, but those instances were indeed rare.

Ward staff complained that the adolescents were destructive, disorganized, almost impossible to manage; in short, they had far too much energy and impulse drive to be able to adjust to life within the confines of a ward.

This picture, obviously, was not much different from that in other state hospitals in the nation, except perhaps for the degree of staff interest and the presence of a number of residents who could offer both individual and group therapy to many of the youngsters. The challenge was clear: to convert a difficult and overwhelming problem—the care and rehabilitation of adolescents —into a constructive, individualized treatment program.

Within two years of the initial report, there was established at Boston State a workable and successful model for the rehabilitation of severely ill hospitalized adolescents, suitable for emulation in large hospitals throughout the country. We shall outline briefly the fundamental features of this imaginative program before describing the process of establishing such a special service.[2]

According to the design set up by the adolescent service, young patients since unitization have been housed on adult wards in the four geographical units. They eat and sleep in these wards, but spend their days in their own center for schooling, recreation, and vocational training. The decision to house the adolescents on the adult wards was a conscious one, based on an intensive analysis of the literature and consultation with many experts in the field. The reports were that when adolescents were treated entirely in their own units, these facilities sooner or later collapsed because of adolescent destruction or severe strain on staff morale.[3] In some all-adolescent units, however, survival is feasible because of a high staff-patient ratio, which was impossible within the budgetary limits of a state hospital. It is also feasible if there were a stringent selection of patients, a policy that was directly counter to the philosophy of the adolescent service as well as that of the administrator.

The core of the treatment program is based on consultation by a small group of trained staff—the adolescent service personnel— to the primary caretakers of adolescents on the wards where they reside. This group serves to stimulate all levels of staff—nurses, social workers, and psychiatric residents—to enter in and maintain therapeutic relationships with their charges. The consultants do not advise on admission policy and firmly resist the tendency of ward staff to hand over the total care of difficult patients to them; instead, they expend their efforts in helping to formulate treatment goals and in coordinating therapeutic actions. As specialists in the treatment of adolescents, they are of distinct help to these primary caretakers in pointing out a latent depression or potential for suicide, an overlooked organic or retardation component, or in sharing their thoughts and knowledge when case dynamics or management is obscure.

Since the central focus of life for most adolescents is school, the service provides two well-staffed facilities: ungraded classes for adolescents with severe learning disabilities and a high school for more capable youngsters, both run by teachers from the Boston school system. Joint correlation of therapeutic with educational activities is part of the service's design. Patients in higher grades remain nominally enrolled in their own local high schools, from which they receive credit for work done at the hospital. Thus, the adolescent receives an unstigmatized diploma, a powerful incentive for those who initially rejected hospital schooling as representing no reward for them.

To encourage adolescents to assume responsibility for their activities, a token reinforcement system was introduced, in which constructive behavior was rewarded with points, applicable to purchases of privileges and extra activities within the adolescent center program. This technique encouraged greater participation by the patients and proved successful in conditioning more acceptable behavior.

Group meetings are held for family members on a weekly basis by the service social workers. Ward staff are encouraged wherever possible to maintain contact with families and even to undertake, in some instances, family therapy or casework under guidance.

The social-recreational program utilizes largely community volunteers for both jaunts away from the hospital and activities in the service day center. The day center, which is open seven days a week, is furnished with all the accouterments close to an adolescent's heart, from a soda fountain to a billiard table.

In short, the service's approach to the treatment of adolescent psychiatric inpatients is based on consultation to primary caretakers on adult residential wards and a specialized program for the adolescents and their families at the central facilities of the adolescent unit.

Administrative Processes in Developing a Special Service

The administrative strategies employed in the development of any new special service in an institutional setting can be illustrated by the example of the adolescent service. The reader will recall that the establishment of the adolescent unit arose in the context of an acute public need for expanded and better services for young, emotionally disturbed patients. The needs of the adolescent—and especially the emotionally ill adolescent—were very much in the air, a source of great community concern and even potential outrage. We may cite such a social ferment as the first criterion for establishing a new project. The proposed effort must be responsive to a felt and dramatic need that for one reason or another has captured public attention. It is sad but true that the community through its legislative representatives is usually reluctant to grant new appropriations to meet longstanding, unfulfilled, but also undramatized needs, for example, the proper treatment of chronic patients or rehabilitation programs for prisoners. It is prepared, however, or can be convinced, to give new resources to meet problems which, if not new, have at least come into sharp focus. Several factors seem to be related to whether or not a given issue comes into the limelight; in the case of adolescents, it is the great human appeal of young people in trouble in a youth-oriented culture. The public is also likely to be responsive to those forms of social pathology that visibly affect them, as does the increased crime rate, drug addiction, and the flagrant forms of deviance that mark our emotionally disturbed young.

We may add here, parenthetically, that the administrator must be prepared to withstand criticism that he is just going where the money is. The accusation is true. Although it is his job to educate the public about other less dramatic, but equally insidious, problems, he cannot pass up any opportunity to do good *now*, to strike while the iron is hot. When the need is so great in all sectors, an administrator cannot afford the luxury of being a Don Quixote. From many concerns, he must select and concentrate on those that resonate to widespread public interest.

The preceding implies our second criterion for the development of a new project. In addition to public demand for action, there must also be ferment within the institution and beginnings of

concerted action prior to the addition of any new outside resources. In the case of the adolescent service, the rising concern
about the fate of young patients had been publicized widely
within the hospital. In addition, the administrator had freed a
social worker's time to investigate the range and depth of the
adolescent problem as it existed at Boston State. It may seem
obvious to stress the administrative importance of this step, yet,
as we noted earlier, it is often extremely difficult to convince a
burdened and service-oriented staff of the wisdom of allowing a
valuable worker to devote her time to such a survey.

We would like to underline that the energy and forcefulness
an administrator must summon to accomplish such an end is one
of the most important aspects of his role. Such a decision may
necessitate some very unpleasant scenes with a department head
or with staff. It is not the kind of decision that can be reached by
a vote. Moreover, some staff are likely to remind the administrator of other such special uses of personnel's time that led to
nothing. But he must persist in following up leads that may pay
off in a sizeable increment to the hospital's total resources. He
must continually educate staff that such an allocation of scarce
personnel may in the long run provide far more service than
would have been accomplished if they just "minded the store."

In thinking about developing the adolescent service, we also
had to keep in mind a third criterion for many new proposed
projects. The program would have to have a demonstration quality; that is, we would be experimenting with new ways of handling
adolescent patients that should have application to their treatment in other state hospitals. If such a program were to be
feasible for widespread use, it obviously could not be an expensive
operation, although it would doubtless entail some additional
resources.

How clear does one have to be about one's program before
seeking such additional outside resources? The answer depends
in part upon the source from which funds are sought. In applying
for a federal demonstration grant, for example, one must be a
great deal clearer than if one is planning to request the conver-

sion of some unused hospital positions into new ones to hire a small staff for a special project. Conversely, the state of one's own thinking and development should be a guide as to where one applies for funds. In the case of the adolescent service, by the end of the survey we knew more clearly the need, but the best ways to meet it were still quite undefined. Information we had obtained led us to believe that it would not be wise to establish a special ward unless it could be densely staffed, which was highly impractical. But beyond this, our ideas were quite undifferentiated. Indeed, it would have been of little help had they been highly specific, since the central lineaments of the program would have to be developed by the still unhired director and staff of the special project. In other words, what we did know was that a substantial treatment program in this important and largely uncharted area would require selected, experienced staff with a special interest in working with the young. The success of the program would above all depend on their enthusiasm, their ideas, their skills, and not ours. Nor would we have the time or special commitment and grass-roots, firsthand knowledge to build up the unit or sustain its quality. Progress in developing the service after its initial start would depend primarily on the unit's ability to attract more resources.

Given the need to establish a beachhead to be occupied initially by a few trained people who could continue and expand the venture, our next practical step was to take the simplest, quickest, and most direct route for new resources. Our initial request from the state was not for new funds, since these must go through a complicated legislative process. What we did ask was that current unused monies for unfilled attendant positions be converted into salaries for a psychiatrist and a psychologist specifically designated to work with adolescents. In short, we wanted to get leaders as quickly as possible who could then take a variety of steps of their own choosing to develop the unit still further.

Incidentally, we might mention that we did not apply for a position for a social worker at this time. Rather, we indicated that as an earnest of the hospital's commitment to the new adolescent service we would keep the same social worker who had conducted the initial survey involved in the new unit. The administrative details are not important. What is significant is that the hospital must commit part of its own resources to get new ones.

Although we have described the conversion of unused positions as the simplest way to providing leadership posts for the proposed unit, this step in practice was by no means easy. In fact, it took almost a year of repeated requests to the state personnel office before success was achieved, and then only after several pressure sources were activated to bear down on that office. These included citizens representing a community organization, a state senator from the hospital area, and the chairman of the hospital board of trustees and his powerful political friends. The problem was that such requests had to meet the criterion of emergency need and that they were vital either to save lives or to save money for the state. We quoted liberally from the social worker's report that "ten to fifteen per cent of the chronic hospital population had entered Boston State as adolescents from ten to as much as fifty years before." In other words, through our failure to supply sufficient treatment for our young patients, we were condemning many of them to lifelong hospitalization.

It should be emphasized that the administrator must proceed carefully in such an instance as just described. He must first have clearly established the priority importance of the request to be made. He cannot constantly run to state officials with "emergency" demands lest he become known as the one who cries wolf all the time. Once he has established the priority of need, he must be prepared to fight on in the face of initial refusal, even if it means mobilizing diverse kinds of support to help him.

Much of the current criticism of the unresponsiveness of large bureaucracies is only partly valid. They *can* be moved to respond —and without tumultuous confrontations—if dramatic need is demonstrated and if persistence with wide support is steadily maintained.

Thus, we finally obtained the two new high-level positions for a psychiatrist and a psychologist. Our next task was also not easy:

to fill these positions with topflight people. In the meantime, our social worker occupied herself with further planning, mobilizing resources, and getting some activity programs for adolescents under way. It was important administratively to keep the momentum of concern about adolescent patients going, being careful at the same time not to create so developed a program that our future psychiatric director would find himself locked into a treatment design not of his own making. What became apparent early through the social worker's efforts was the highly favorable response on the part of staff and volunteers to working on a project specially devoted to adolescents. Chronicity, which is above all characterized by an inability to enjoy oneself, to give oneself over to any activity, is sad at any age, but it is especially heartrending to see in the young. Our social worker was particularly adept at using volunteers to provide activities for adolescent patients and this great willingness to utilize all kinds of help continues to characterize the adolescent service.

Our search for a unit chief went on. After considerable screening, we finally found a psychiatrist who met the requirements for this key position. We may pause to describe the administrator's relationship with this young man during the phase of recruitment since it illustrates some concepts that are particularly significant in developing new services.

We stated in chapter 1 that it was important for the administrator to keep and develop contacts with able people outside the institution, not least for purposes of recruitment. The administrator had known this particular psychiatrist since his residency and had maintained regular contact with him over the years. He had high admiration for the psychiatrist's drive, intelligence, and clinical skills and believed he would be an ideal person to head the adolescent service.

Recruiting a high-level person for a new, special service is almost always a delicate process. One must excite the candidate's imagination and give him some idea of the potential scope of the new development. At the same time, one must warn him of the real difficulties of working in a state hospital system, lest he later feel that he has been sold a bill of goods.

In meeting the first part of this equation, the administrator emphasized the freedom our candidate would have in molding a service according to his own vision. However, he also made it very clear that although the unit would have whatever support he could give, it would largely have to muster its staff through its own enterprise in gaining outside grants. It was important that the new director not enter the hospital with any illusions about an abundance of resources suddenly being directed his way. Not only did the real demands of the hospital prevent such a grossly unequal distribution, but it would also have been devastating to the morale of the regular services, which were operating with acute staff shortages.

With a mandate granting considerable freedom, but with his eyes open to the realities of the situation, our candidate became director of the adolescent service.

Let us turn now to the kind of administrative measures the administrator had to take in order to facilitate the development of the adolescent service.

First, it is necessary for the administrator to give a new, enthusiastic director steady and generous initial support as he starts to build an enterprise of his own within a complex, ongoing system. For example, the new director needed office space for himself and his team. The administrator took some pains to make sure that he got such space in a building of his own choosing—the reception building which, prior to unitization, housed most of the adolescent patients. Again, this may sound like a commonplace, garden-variety problem. In fact, however, it necessitated strenuous discussion with the maintenance department to get them to make the necessary renovations and adjustments to provide offices in an already overcrowded building. It is important to note that there are always objections to any effort that must be made to accomodate new people, particularly when they have special wishes that may inconvenience hospital personnel. The steward has his own order of priorities and it takes some administrative persuasion for him to put a new project at the top of his list. Not that he will actually refuse an administrator's request, but he will find all kinds of reasons why the necessary adjustments cannot be made.

In this instance, the administrator was told that there was no money available for lumber for the renovation. Fortunately, the administrator was able to use two hundred dollars from unrestricted funds to overcome that particular resistance.

Quite often, the administrator's support not only entails difficulties with the business office, but also with professional colleagues of the new person, who, indeed, can readily appear to older staff members as a sudden, unwelcome, and favored sibling. In our example, the new man was indeed getting a larger and more comfortable private office than the director of the inpatient service located in that building. The administrator found he had to temper his support, since given in excess it would have unduly jeopardized the morale of regular personnel. Even so, he had constantly to face many criticisms that he was favoring special projects at the cost of the regular inpatient services.

Balancing the claims of new innovative talents against those of the hospital staff as a whole is an extremely complex and often poignant task for the administrator. Yet it is our thesis that he cannot avoid this dilemma by some kind of standardized criteria which most people could easily accept as fair. Nor can he turn decisions about priorities entirely over to some kind of democratic group process. The latter also tends to move toward formal criteria—fair for one, fair for all. In our example, for instance, it is very doubtful that initially, when the new director arrived, the psychiatric executive committee or the senior staff as a whole would have voted to give him special and reconverted space in the crowded reception building.

It may appear contradictory in the light of our earlier arguments for wide participation in decision-making that we are now arguing for the administrator retaining and ultilizing considerable power in the setting of priorities. We do not believe this is an either/or question, but rather that the answer lies in a kind of creative synthesis of the two. Nor can we claim that such a synthesis is anything but fraught with problems.

For example, it may be rightly argued that although an administrator sets priorities, his rationale should be fully discussed. Yet it is very hard to discuss in a public forum that so and so is getting a special favor on a rush basis because he has extraordinary potential and because the service he is heading is in some sense more important than some other service. The adolescent service was only more important in that it was responding to a desperate, dramatic need at the appropriate time. If we gave it unusual support, it could also galvanize unusual further support from the outside because of the great public interest in this area.

The administrator, then, often keeps his cards close to his vest not necessarily because he dislikes explaining his moves to his subordinates but because of his awareness of the heated emotions generated by what is called administrative favoritism. True, the lack of formal discussion does not prevent negative feelings about such administrative decisions; there is always an undercurrent of dissatisfaction on the part of some people. But the reasons are not rubbed in through formal explanation, thus saving face for those not so favored.

We do not make the points just cited because we are against open discussion of administrative decisions. On the contrary, we are for it in most instances. We only wish in this context to stress some of the social dysfunctions of such discussion and to raise certain questions about the feasibility of any mechanical dicta regarding complete openness in decision-making. We need not here elaborate the arguments against administrative secrecy. The obvious one, of course, is that it serves to maintain an authoritarian atmosphere in which "father knows best" and need not explain himself to the children.

Administrative support of the new adolescent unit was not limited to facilitating the creation of office space. We have mentioned earlier that the adolescent unit was designed as a consultation service, as well as a unit that could provide concentrated services, such as education and group activities. Toward both these goals, the unit staff itself was extremely active in building up its own connections, demonstrating its usefulness to other staff and attracting new resources. The administrator's task was mainly one of guidance and support.

We discussed in chapter 1 the importance of the administrator's making an individual diagnosis of each key staff member and giving administrative therapy if necessary. Such close concern is especially significant with new persons embarking on important ventures. We can perhaps illustrate what we mean by describing in more detail the administrator's continuing relationship with the adolescent service director. The administrator recognized early that he would need considerable and ongoing support. Ideas and initiative he would have in abundance, but his tolerance for disappointment would have to be watched. More or less informally it worked out that the two met regularly once a week in the beginning months. This gave him a chance to ventilate his frustrations in consulting with recalcitrant ward staff about difficult cases or in obtaining needed resources. With regard to the latter, the administrator was frequently reminded of the wisdom of his earlier strong communication to the new director that he would have to attract these resources from outside agencies. In the course of the talks, it was important to show a steady interest, backed up by prompt and energetic steps wherever the administrator could be helpful.

The new director was remarkably successful in negotiating with a wide variety of institutions for additional help. Thus he was able over a few years to increase the original complement of two teachers to seven, all paid by the city government. The administrator's task here was to help him face some original disappointments when early requests were refused or bottled up, and to encourage his own inclination to keep pressing toward his goal. In other instances, help could be more substantial, for example, by strengthening the research aspect of a proposal which eventually led to a substantial federal grant and an increase in the original unit staff.

But citing particular measures does not delineate fully the intricate issues in dealing with high-energy creative persons leading innovative projects. The problems of working with such people are frequently just the opposite from those encountered in dealing with regular members of the hospital. It is not a question of urging and propelling them to start or expand programs, to look to other institutions for new ideas, or of lifting them out of well-worn ruts. Rather, it is a question of helping them tolerate the inevitable disappointments and delays in accomplishing anything worthwhile—obstacles sorely aggravated in a state hospital setting. It is helping them learn to get along with persons whose aid is indispensable but who are often not so fast moving as they, or who are resistive to the new man with the bright ideas.

The special-unit people were often extremely critical of regular staff members whom they deemed rigid, unimaginative, or incompetent. The administrator had sometimes to restrain their anger at accustomed ways of doing things or even more to resist their urging that he be firm with this one or that one. Sometimes, their critical energies could be constructively channeled. He encouraged one such person to voice many of his complaints, particularly on the education of personnel, at some of our seniors' meetings. This was helpful in bringing certain issues to attention without provoking the resistances that arise when such criticism comes from the administrator.

Just as it was important to meet many of the demands of persons starting special projects, so it was important to set limits on what they could gain. Whereas many regular employees assiduously avoid the top administrator, or are afraid to approach him, high-energy persons with a mandate for starting new programs usually try to corner him to enlist his aid. The administrator grew accustomed to seeing them waiting for him on his arrival in the morning or trying to catch him for a few minutes at the end of the day. The administrator's open-door policy facilitated this kind of communication and such persons had the temperament to take full advantage of it. It is essential to wean these activists gradually from so close a relationship with the administrator. It is equally essential for several reasons to permit a good deal of it in the initial phases of their enterprise. First, they often need massive support during the difficult beginning days, just as a new arrival in the family needs special care during his most vulnerable years of growth. Second, as we have also mentioned, their demands in the early days are often difficult to justify in public places. If the administrator can quietly help them during the period of growing up without bringing down too much wrath from their peers, they can fight their own battles for resources after they have obtained some initial success.

As an illustration, once the adolescent service had demonstrated on its own its usefulness to the hospital and had acquired considerable outside funds, staff as a whole was much more tolerant of the service's obtaining still further hospital resources. Private negotiations between special-unit director and the administrator were no longer necessary.

The issue might readily be raised at this point that all the units —old as well as new, regular as well as special—would have benefitted from the close attention time allowed the administrator to give to only some of them. Undoubtedly, he gave more attention to some new projects because he thought their particular characteristics would generate further help once they got off the ground. But, in addition, he gave the help because it was sought and even more because it was fruitfully used. On other occasions he tried to enliven a particular discipline or a particular area of the hospital through taking the initiative in giving support and resources. On some occasions, such action was not particularly successful. The help was seen as only small relief for an overwhelming need. It did not generate further activity, which in turn could have elicited further help both from the administrator and from others.

In short, then, an administrator makes certain bets initially with the relatively small resources at his disposal. He makes them on complex grounds, not easily made explicit in terms of prototypal criteria. In a sense he functions like a bank giving a loan, subtly appraising the potential of the new enterprise. To continue our metaphor, if the loan pays off, it is now much easier to show through the balance sheet of the new company that it needs and deserves another loan for further expansion.

In the case of the adolescent service, the administrator began with the initial investment of a social worker's time to make a survey of the needs of adolescent patients. Armed with this information, he took the next small but significant investment of trading vacant, nonprofessional positions for professional ones. The risk element here was not so much the loss of the attendant positions, but the decision to use some of the reservoir of good will from various influential persons to exercise pressure for the administrative conversion. His next investment was the considerable time and special attention given to the adolescent service in its initial phases of development. These particular risks paid off. The original investment of a social worker's time led within a few years to a large staff trained in the care and treatment of adolescents operating on a large budget funded in good part by outside agencies. The unit not only significantly improved the treatment of adolescent patients but also, through the conscientious supervision and sophisticated consultation it provided to staff members, it became a crucial resource indirectly benefitting many adult patients.

REFERENCES

1. B. A. Glasser, "Parental Attitudes Toward the Hospital Experience," in *Adolescents in a Mental Hospital,* ed. E. Hartmann et al. (New York: Grune and Stratton, 1968), pp. 62–69; B. A. Glasser, E. Hartmann, and N. C. Avery, "Attitudes Toward Adolescents on Adult Wards of a Mental Hospital," *American Journal of Psychiatry* 124 (1967): 317–22.

2. A. O. Kris and L. F. Schiff, "An Adolescent Consultation Service in a State Mental Hospital: Maintaining Treatment Motivation," *Seminars in Psychiatry* 1 (1969): 15–23.

3. H. Beskind, "Psychiatric Inpatient Treatment of Adolescents: A Review of Clinical Experience," *Comprehensive Psychiatry* 3 (1962): 354–69.

CHAPTER 6

The Rehabilitation Service

In the preceding chapter we discussed the development of a special unit that had two distinct advantages. For one, it served a group of patients for whom staff felt considerable interest and sympathy—adolescents. For the other, its strong emphasis on psychotherapy was shared by most of the professional staff. In this chapter we shall be concerned with the evolution of another new service, rehabilitation, or work therapy, which was primarily focused on a group of patients toward whom staff held pessimistic attitudes—chronically ill, apathetic, and defeated middle-aged men and women. In addition, the emphasis that was to be placed on work as a treatment modality represented a radical shift in thinking and one that staff could accomodate themselves to only with stress and conflict.

Some of the administrative problems to be discussed will concern the organizational issues that arise in the course of a basic, sharp, and affect-laden ideological conflict between the concept of work as therapy advanced by the administrator and the traditional ways of thinking represented by the majority of the hospital staff.

Work Therapy at Boston State in 1963

At most large mental hospitals, free patient labor constitutes a considerable part of the hospital work force; at Boston State, for example, patients had rendered the equivalent of half a million dollars of services during 1963 alone. This figure is less surprising when one realizes that a hospital serving twenty-four hundred patients on a relatively low budget must, in many ways, take care of its own service tasks. It does not, for example, send out its sheets, towels, patients' clothes, and uniforms to the local linen service. The hospital has its own laundry, and the chronic shortage of paid employees often means that many patients must work in that facility.

The following incident was typical of the system when the administrator first arrived: A laundry worker would call up a male ward and say "I need eleven workers or I can't get your laundry out." The nurse on duty would quickly select eleven men and send them along. Some patients went willingly, others reluctantly, but most often coercion was necessary. Some liked the job; others merely tolerated it. Some did well; others scarcely pulled their weight. The same applied to patients (about 17 percent of the population) working in other hospital jobs—shipping, dishwashing, sewing, gardening, snow-shoveling, plumbing, and so on.

For the great majority of these patients, work was therapy only by accident. Basically, they were assigned to any work area that was short of help, without full assessment of their occupational history or work capacity and without sufficient consideration of the relationship between the work expected from them and their emotional problems. Rarely was there consultation with the patient's psychiatrist. Good workers were jealously guarded by hard-pressed hospital employees; discharge of any one of them to the community was a loss. One can readily see how the work system militated against the return to the community of precisely those patients, the good workers, who might do best outside the hospital.

Thus, although it was undoubtedly better for most patients to be occupied rather than to sit idly on the wards, nothing could disguise the fact that the system was a form of institutional peonage. Patients worked in some thirty to forty hospital areas, the vast majority without a cent of pay. To the work supervisors, they were a special breed—a cross between a favorite pet and a slave laborer. Some treated them with kindness; others were domineering and authoritarian. In any case, the supervisors mainly kept their eye on what was good for their service or industry. They rarely considered themselves as part of the therapeutic team and, in fact, were rarely included in any kind of clinical evaluation or systematic instruction in the therapeutic potential of their roles.

There were, however, some rewards to the patients: the relief in getting off the ward with its empty tedium; the satisfaction of being active in producing a tangible commodity; the belonging to a familiar group, even if communication was minimal; and the pleasing of one's boss, rewarded often by a smile, a kind word, or a package of cigarettes. Some patients were uniquely able to profit by these conditions and did in fact improve. But too many became arrested in their chronicity: supervisor and patient had settled for a tacit contract that implied, "You do what I tell you; I won't put further demands on you." Thus, instead of a truly therapeutic program with progressive, realistic, organized steps and expectations, and with appropriate aids to negotiate impasses, the system was geared to maintaining the hospital's various service departments.

The arrangement just described reflected a lack of any value on work as therapy. There was no department of rehabilitation as such; all work programming was administered by a small department of occupational therapy, which emphasized manual diversions for regressed patients rather than supervised and practical work experience. The whole work program was peripheral to the main interest of the occupational therapist, and an extra load at that.

Philosophy of Work Therapy

The reader may ask why psychiatry in America has neglected, indeed often resisted, involvement in programs of work therapy. It would appear that the profession has been too preoccupied with exploring the intricacies of psychological processes in mental disease and in treating emotional disorder by dynamic psychotherapy. Its concentration has been on psychopathology rather than on the skills and assets patients possess that can be activated with proper encouragement.

It is true that recent developments in ego psychology have opened up the possibility of work being viewed as a therapeutic modality. However, ego psychology seems to hold less fascination for the average psychiatrist, particularly the beginner, than delving into unconscious processes. The occasional remarkable improvements reported in chronic patients through work therapy have been either glossed over or explained away as a product of the strong transference relationship that the patient was fortunately able to develop toward his work supervisor or some other helpful individual. Since there are few well-developed theoretical models to explain the efficacy of work therapy, perhaps the reader will forgive us if we attempt a few tentative speculations.

Man was not made to be idle. He was given eyes to see his prey or attacker, ears to hear danger, a nose to sniff trouble, strong musculature to pursue or flee an opponent, and a digestive apparatus to bite, chew, swallow, and assimilate his fuel for life. His autonomic nervous system mobilizes his visceral apparatus for fight or flight—or for rest, recuperation, or reproduction.

With the passage of eons of history, man emerges in modern times as a worker instead of a marauder, a producer of goods or services to be exchanged for food and shelter, rather than a hunter. But, the same expenditure of energy in eye, muscle, and sinew must alternate with periods of restoration as in ancient times. If this cycle is broken through withdrawal from activity, man's coping mechanisms fall into disuse, and the doing-resting rhythm becomes a flat line of apathy, indolence, and tedium.

Work that fits the individual's basic personality needs gives both pleasure and gratification. There is the satisfaction in seeing the useful product develop and take shape; and the knowledge that it can be applied to better living for himself or others can be ego-strengthening. The mastery of a skill that yields goods needed by others makes the person a man among men.

The meaning of a specific type of work activity or job derives in considerable measure from an individual's past relationships. Thus, because his mother showed extraordinary interest in fabrics, the son became a successful mill owner. Or a son chooses medicine as a career because his father is a physician who enjoys his work and extols its virtues to his family. In many much more subtle and symbolic ways the work represents an introjected aspect of a significant emotional tie to an important other. Thus it can be said that behind every job, and even within the relationships between man and the machine that is his means of production, lies the representation of some earlier relationship.

Thus, work is an emotionally and biologically complex and significant function of man; as such it deserves as much attention from the modern psychiatrist as the patient's inner life, his family, or his dreams.

However, not only the psychiatrist's theoretical bias in favor of highly specific psychological and somatic treatments, but also his own vocational, social, and educational experiences isolate him from the work world of the average state hospital patient. He knows little about the jobs that lower-class patients are used to, from which they will have to earn a living when they return to the community. Many psychiatrists, in fact, are frankly uninterested in such activities as working in a laundry, kitchen, or factory. They are much less concerned about the ways a patient's functioning could be improved through such manual work or with the way his psychodynamic problems interfere with competent job performance than they are with, for example, the importance of helping a college dropout master his work problems so he can return to school.

It requires, then, a concerted effort for many professionals to take a serious and empathic look at how work—often blue-collar and at best low-grade white-collar work—can serve the therapeutic interests of the patient. They argue that work often serves the interest of the hospital rather than the patient, and can be used by staff to avoid dealing with the patient's illness. Our quarrel is not with these arguments themselves, but with the fact that their proponents use them for negative purposes. They are not concerned with improving the work program so that it *can* serve the patient rather than the hospital, but with making certain that work does not interfere with traditional psychotherapeutic activities.

However, if our thoughts about the psychological meaning of work have any validity, a great deal of good could flow from proper organization of work programs. We could say categorically that in the mental hospital, as we have known it, work therapy is in general at *least* as potent a treatment as any other modality in use.

Establishing a Work Program

In the previous chapter the weight of the administrator's personal and administrative support for new persons undertaking innovative projects was stressed. In a sense, the administrator must, to use an analogy, give the proper drugs to help combat the organismic rejection of a foreign body. In the case of the rehabilitation service, the administrator had to introduce not only new persons but also some foreign and unappealing ideas and to help defend both against the rejection mechanism.

Since there was no group at the hospital specially devoted to work therapy, and since the administrator placed a high value on such treatment, it was essential that he put the program into the hands of a separate group of specialists in rehabilitation and to make that service answerable directly to central administration. Experience with other efforts showed that new programs and new ideas can be quickly crushed by the inertia and resistance of middle management if department heads are not fully committed to their value. The top administrator must often assume responsibility for new and resisted enterprises even at the risk of overloading his office with extra burdens.

One of the first administrative steps was to establish a new position: a rehabilitation coordinator. To accomplish this, we used an unfilled post in the occupational therapy department as our initial "risk capital" for the rehabilitation venture. Fortunately, we were able to recruit from a neighboring hospital that had pioneered in work therapy a rehabilitation counselor who had utilized Boston State as a training site for students, since his own institution lacked long-term patients. In recruiting him, we gained: (1) his extensive knowledge of the rehabilitation problems at the hospital, and (2) the help of students who had worked with him. In addition, in the early stages we employed as consultant a man who had developed an outstanding work therapy program at still another state hospital.

In establishing any new program, it is essential to engage energetic and dedicated specialists particularly if the enterprise needs more than usual development. The administrator will err if, in order to court acceptance of the program by hospital personnel, he limits himself to recruiting only from the ranks and is saddled with individuals with less than superior talent, interest, and expertise. In the case of rehabilitation, our task in recruiting skilled work therapists was made somewhat easier by the relatively low esteem in which the art was held elsewhere. We found that counselors from other institutions welcomed the opportunity to work, even if with some job insecurity, in a setting where administration valued work therapy highly and was prepared to support it vigorously.

The next administrative step was to encourage the rehabilitation coordinator, the consultant, and the student assistants to transmit the philosophy of rehabilitation to various supervisors of work areas. Few of these work supervisors imagined that anyone would want them to become part of a therapeutic team. It took a great deal of convincing, as the efforts described by one work therapist indicate:

You have to be willing to stand in the grease pool in the garage, address the mechanic and say, "Look, what do *you* think are the patient's needs?" and, by constant seeking of their advice and judgment, bring them into the treatment group. It means inviting to staff meetings people wearing cafeteria uniforms, carpenter outfits, aprons greasy from a plumbing job, or overalls smelling of garden fertilizer.

This rehabilitation counselor further described the first hospital staff conference held with a work supervisor:

I invited a fellow from the grounds crew to our staff meeting. He didn't know what it was. "What do you want me there for? Did I do something wrong?" I said, "I want you to talk about a patient you've been working with." He thought I was kidding. "Who's gonna be there? Do I have to get clearance from my department head?" I said I would arrange clearance on everything.

He came to the staff meeting directly from work—dirty and unshaven. I introduced him and asked him to comment on the patient working with him. He looked frightened, but the respect given him by "the professionals" encouraged him to loosen up. He talked in simple language—often using four-letter words—consistent with his education and upbringing: a former boxer, a rough, tough guy.

He was giving his opinion about a patient he knew better than anyone else and people respected his knowledge by asking him, "Should he work more hours? Could he do that job in the community?" This was the first time anyone had ever asked his advice or opinion. He began to have a new concept of himself and felt that he was contributing something to the welfare of the patient.

This same work therapist eventually came to the conviction that the heart of the rehabilitation program rested with the kinds of relationships the counselors were able to establish with such line supervisors,[1] for it was the latter who provided the actual work therapy for the patient, who had the firsthand knowledge of the patient's capacities and problems, and who were in a position to provide the matrix of instruction, encouragement, and criticism to develop the patient as an independent worker.

Another key administrative step was to develop programs for paid employment of patients. To the administrator it was morally unacceptable for a state hospital to depend on the unpaid help of its patients who, if not for the nature of their illness, could band together to assert their demands. There was in fact a law on the books of the commowealth that patients working in a state mental hospital should receive compensation, but funds were never voted and hence nothing was implemented. Once again, it was necessary to work around and outside the system in order to meet a goal few could quarrel with in principle.

Prior to the administrator's coming to Boston State, Dr. Barton had already taken a pioneering step in developing a small paid patient-employee program (PEP) which rewarded certain patients with sixteen dollars per week for their work. It was stipulated, however, that this money was to be used only to help those who could be expected to enter community employment within a reasonably short time. Unfortunately, since there were not enough able staff to man an active rehabilitation program which would include prevocational training, only the relatively few patients who were *already* competent in terms of work could make use of PEP.

Thus, it was necessary not only to raise more money to pay patients for work of all kinds, but also to provide the vocational counseling and clinical supervision that would permit them to take maximum advantage of a program such as PEP. It became increasingly clear that this kind of clinical push in the work area required closer day-to-day psychiatric leadership and inspiration than the administrator, personally, was in a position to provide.

We were fortunate in being able to share a considerable part of the burden of developing the rehabilitation program with the newly appointed assistant superintendent. This psychiatrist brought to the challenge many talents: a longstanding interest in rehabilitation, an unusual ability to communicate with lower-level personnel, and a capacity to maintain the steady pressure so necessary for this new project. Also, by virtue of his professional role and the fact that he had top-level administrative support, he was in an excellent position to handle the resistance he was bound to encounter. It was important that a highly visible top-echelon psychiatrist should stand for work rehabilitation to help bridge the gap between the realm of work and the realm of psychiatric practice.

(A side aspect of this appointment is germane to the issue of administration in general. We mentioned in chapter 1 that the position of assistant superintendent can often be routine and uninspiring. To give such a person broad, semiautonomous responsibility in a new, tough domain not only makes good use of his administrative leverage, but also helps him carve a role that is far more fulfilling than that of the traditional vice-president.)

To fortify the program, the assistant superintendent made special efforts to recruit professionals who evinced some interest in work therapy. Thus, one psychiatric resident, who was singular among his colleagues in this respect, joined a PEP clinical team to help provide the evaluation, supervision, and screening the program lacked. The superintendent, as well as the assistant superintendent, gave administrative backing to this somewhat unorthodox deployment of a second-year resident. Still another professional addition was a distinguished physician, not a psychiatrist, with a long interest in physical as well as psychiatric rehabilitation. He was slipped into an unfilled junior staff position.

The above two instances may be worth a moment's digression: Not only was it unusual to have a resident involved in such a program, but it was also unusual, to say the least, to utilize a vacant post for a junior psychiatrist to hire a physician with a distinguished career in physical medicine. We wish to underline that: (1) by and large, one cannot build up a new department in a traditional way in a state hospital, and (2) one must often begin with makeshift arrangements pieced together from here and there. It is the use of pay blocks as "risk capital" in unusual and unorthodox ways (sometimes to the chagrin of state-level personnel officers) that may spell the difference between success or failure in new and nontraditional programs.

Our next major step was directed toward setting up sheltered workshops in the hospital. We hoped these would help patients develop their vocational skills, without being restricted by the fiscal and employment regulations of the PEP program. We knew that the necessary resources for paid employment of a substantial number of patients would have to come from outside. Our rehabilitation coordinator believed he could obtain contracts from the garment industry, but lacked the money to buy sewing machines, the basic equipment for a workshop. The administrator suggested that he discuss the situation with a successful, dynamic business executive he knew, who wanted to do something for people less fortunate than he. This man not only agreed to meet the initial request but also promised to collaborate with the hospital in setting up a series of model contract workshops where patients could be paid and where the workshops would be an essential link in a total rehabilitation enterprise.[2] He instinctively understood the problems of working with the mentally disabled and he possessed the business acumen, the wide circle of contacts, and the organizational genius to give the work program a tremendous boost. His contribution and those of his associates exemplified the remarkable potential of state hospital collaboration with experienced, hardheaded, knowledgeable men of the business world.

These men laid the foundation for PROP, Inc. (Patient Rehabilitation Occupation Program). In their design, with which we fully agreed, PROP would solicit contracts, raise funds, provide extra consultation, renovate quarters, and install equipment. The hospital in turn would provide space, give what staff it could muster for the work program, and continue to supply all other services necessary for a comprehensive rehabilitation service. Under this aegis, the workshop grew within a few months from a small enterprise containing three sewing machines to a plant containing forty of them, all in active use. A pressing service and assembly shop were added in a short time, and a printing plant was set up in a contiguous building. The men behind PROP got their friends and business associates to give year-round contracts to help keep the shops—which soon became a beehive of activity for about eighty patients—busy.

Work activities were organized along the lines of a regular factory. Patients were exposed to the many situations they might find in private industry, from time-clock punching to appropriate dress. They were paid by check, the payer being the company from which the work was contracted, not the hospital. Money was deposited in the bank and could be withdrawn at will, unless a patient's doctor intervened for good cause. Each patient was allowed to accumulate a nest egg of several hundred dollars;

thereafter, he paid a percentage of his earnings to the hospital for room and board. In a word, he earned his own money and began to pay his own way. By this means, we were reversing the pattern of giving the chronic patient little and expecting even less in return.

About one of every four patients involved in the work program was able to obtain community employment within four or five months; some took a little longer. But even for those who were unable to make the grade, living was much better in the hospital if they were employed. Working seemed to elevate their badly damaged senses of dignity, self-esteem, and self-worth. And little wonder: some patients had neither worked nor earned money for the twenty or thirty long years they had been hospitalized.

Thus, PROP meant a major additional influx of community resources, the kind of infusion from without that a state hospital needs so desperately. This infusion consisted not only of money and skilled supervision, but also involved the tangible components of drive, flexibility, and resourcefulness that the businessmen exhibited, setting a needed example for many hospital employees mired in routine.

Furthermore, the businessmen's interest and help gave a great lift to the morale of the entire rehabilitation department. We have mentioned that the typical professional was not especially enthusiastic about work therapy. The rehabilitation service, like other departments, needed sustenance and support from outside groups. Just as the researcher looked to academic colleagues at other institutions as an important source of encouragement and support, so the work therapist looked to industry as one of his reference groups.

In review, the initial rehabilitation cadre of one coordinator and one consultant had helped to stimulate interest in work therapy among many supervisors of patient-workers. The assistant superintendent helped enlist, through his enthusiasm and commitment, the cooperation of several physicians in the work program. The introduction of PROP brought new vocational training sites and paid employment for a substantial number of patients. However, the rehabilitation program still lacked a sufficient number of well-trained counselors who could work closely with, and have a real impact on, the regular hospital ward staff.

To meet this need, we applied for and received a federal hospital improvement grant. This grant enhanced the whole rehabilitation enterprise, providing as it did the means to add several counselors. Prior to the grant, the work therapy forces, though scattered and limited, had created a separate department, joining forces with a few occupational therapists and the head of the industrial therapy program. Even with the incorporation of PROP staff, the department still represented a centralized service. However, with the addition of the new counselors under the grant, it was possible to decentralize the operation and to assign work therapists to the four basic inpatient units to plan rehabilitation programs with the ward teams.

This kind of decentralization, following a period of centralization, represents a crucial organizational rhythm of new projects. Whether the program is initially funded by an outside grant, or, as in the case of the rehabilitation service, is a patchwork structure built up from scattered, existing positions and activities, their forces must be consolidated in the early phases. Thus, through collective strength, appropriate strategies can be planned to achieve specified goals and to attract new resources from the community. Some aspects of new programs must remain centralized in order to coordinate functions throughout the institution, but often at the cost of being psychologically isolated from the rest of the hospital. The staff of the new service will continue to be seen as "them"—outsiders and strangers—by the regular hospital personnel, who have the overall responsibility for the patients. This indeed happened, to some extent, with the rehabilitation service. As long as it remained centralized, it had to continually "sell itself," to seek out patient referrals. Occasionally, ward staff might spontaneously get in touch with the rehabilitation people if they had an ideal patient who could very clearly benefit from a work program. But they were just as apt to refer the least-likely-to-succeed patient—a hostile referral.

The day-to-day dialogue in which rehabilitation and ward personnel could exchange views, appreciate each other's talents, and be fully useful to patients did not *really* occur until counselors were assigned to units and spent considerable time there. Many of the work therapists were part of a unit team and could be considered by each unit as belonging to "us," rather than to an undifferentiated, distant, grant-rich and privileged research elite.

We may add, parenthetically, that this healthy centralization-decentralization sequence is more likely to occur when the new program, such as the rehabilitation or the adolescent service, does *not* have overall responsibility for a group of patients. The consultative nature of the task the new program's staff face necessitates their assigning particular people to particular in-patient units and thus developing close relationships with ward staff. If, on the other hand, a new demonstration project has its own case load—alcoholics or drug addicts, for example—and complete responsibility for them, it tends to remain isolated from the rest of the hospital. The experience it acquires is shared only very slowly, if at all, with the regular inpatient units, who often have to deal with similar patients, but in a much less specialized setting.

Obstacles and Clashes

A program strongly backed by administration but not highly valued by the rest of the hospital is bound to run into difficulty. This was particularly true in the case of the rehabilitation service, which attempted to mobilize all hospital staff, from ward personnel to working area people, to share in what many believed was an unjustified enthusiasm for work therapy.

One initial difficulty was jurisdictional. Whenever a new department is introduced that is closely allied, operationally and conceptually, to another department, the established department is likely to feel that its territory had been invaded. In the case of the rehabilitation service, the most closely allied services were occupational therapy and social work. Although, as mentioned, the occupational therapists had oriented themselves primarily to providing recreational activities for patients and only secondarily to the work program, they still resented the creation of a new department that intended to develop an area for which they already had some responsibility. In this instance, the initial frictions were resolved by both groups quite successfully through a division of labor; the occupational therapists took responsibility for assessing the vocational capacities of patients and the rehabilitation service took charge of actual supervision of ongoing work therapy.

Whereas the responsibilities of occupational therapy and rehabilitation overlapped in the area of developing work skills, the responsibilities of rehabilitation and social work overlapped in placing patients in community employment. In actual fact, the chronic shortage of social workers meant that the amount of intensive job placement they could do was very limited. However, the social workers tended to feel superior to the new breed of work therapists and never effectively joined forces with them. They believed that the rehabilitation people should be incorporated into the social work department, but in a subordinate position. Particular personalities aside, it does seem easier for a new department to join forces with persons who do not see themselves as professionally superior to the "invaders" but who sense, rather, that through collaboration their own role definition will become clearer and their prestige heightened.

In the early phases, then, while the rehabilitation service was still an organizational infant, its main struggles were essentially with the paramedical rather than the medical departments of the hospital, which stayed aloof, too important to quarrel with anything quite so insignificant. The attitude of many of the medical staff was well expressed by the following anecdote, related to us by a work therapist:

In the beginning there were an awful lot of psychiatric staff who had no idea what we were doing. In fact, one of the things that happened was that I got a call one day from the wife of a physician living on the hospital grounds, complaining, "My refrigerator is broken." I said, "Why are you calling me?" "Well," she said, "I understand you fix things." I answered, "Yes, but that's not what I fix." I began to wonder, then, what I *was* doing, if that was her image of me.

However, as work therapy grew, and particularly after the inclusion of some maverick physicians, the psychiatric staff, in general, no longer ignored the service, but became actively irritated with it. This was especially true when the rehabilitation service began to flex its muscles and assert its rights over the patients' time. Psychiatrists saw no reason why work therapy should be considered as important as individual or group psychotherapy. Residents had made elaborate plans to invest at least a full year in the psychotherapy of a chronic patient, and consultants were being paid good money to give individual supervision on a once-a-week basis. Once the hours of therapy and supervision were arranged, it was extremely disruptive to be asked to alter the program because a rehabilitation worker, with no special commitment to psychotherapy, wanted the patient's work day to be considered inviolate. If the young resident went to the director of psychiatry and asked, "Who is going to see the patient at eleven—the rehab man or me?" the boat truly began to rock.

Friction was also inevitable with others involved in the total care of the patient. To quote a rehabilitation counselor:

We asked the podiatrist to change appointments so patients could have their feet treated after work; we asked the barber if he could cut a patient's hair in the morning or on a Saturday; we asked volunteers who were taking patients out during their best working hours to change the excursions to evenings or weekends. We had to sit down with everyone interested in the patient to work out an individual plan so that, let's say, psychotherapy could be given first thing in the morning or dentist appointments scheduled for the late afternoon.

Often frictions could be settled amicably in this round-table fashion, but sometimes the clashes were of such magnitude that the administrator was called in to intervene. In general, he tried to avoid laying down a specific decree. Rather, he stressed his general philosophy that he valued work therapy highly, on a par with individual or group psychotherapy, and that its results with chronic patients were both practical and tangible. On the other hand, he sometimes had to curb the enthusiasm of the work therapists, who were inclined to minimize completely the legitimate needs of the resident training program.

Another way he tried to strengthen the rehabilitation program was to reward those persons whose own commitment was in line with the evolving orientation of work therapy. This was particularly important in the case of medical staff. For example, he took great pains to support a fourth-year resident whose interest in psychopharmacology had led to his working with chronic patients; over time, he became greatly interested in the possibilities of work therapy with these same patients. The energy he gave to this task and the success he had with very long-term patients lent a prestige to rehabilitation within the hospital community that could not be gained through similar efforts by nonmedical personnel. Thus, it often takes interest by medical leadership to give a hospital program real gusto.

The rehabilitation service clashed not only with medical and paramedical personnel, but with work-area employees as well. Programs of paid work, such as PEP and PROP, were viewed by many maintenance people as a drain from much needed, but unpaid, hospital labor. Moreover, the very fact that some patients were being paid made other patients object to working unless they too were reimbursed. The increase in paid work programs also occurred at a time when the census was being reduced, thereby depleting overall manpower for *any* kind of labor. For a variety of reasons, then, the basic hospital services, which depended heavily on unpaid labor, were suffering and it was only natural for them to blame "that newfangled work program."

Even when the rehabilitation department did help to find and supervise labor attached to the unpaid hospital industries, the resistances of line supervisors were manifold. As pointed out, some felt pleased to be included in clinical discussions, but many either felt threatened or simply did not want to be bothered. Just as the work therapy program was viewed by the clinical staff as too "grubby," so it was viewed by the maintenance people as too "clinical." If, by chance, a line worker did become interested in work therapy, his department head often resented his spending time attending conferences about patients. Some supervisors also felt that unless the patients were really capable, it was wasting the employee's time to teach them. Still other work-area employees felt that they were not paid to help patients, but to do their particular jobs.

The rehabilitation department, then, was trying to effect a marriage between two equally unwilling partners—the professionals and the maintenance people. In so doing, it was running right into a kind of cleavage that divides most large hospitals. Professionals are viewed with great ambivalence by persons concerned with the organizational innards of an institution—the kitchen, the garage, the laundry. Maintenance is staffed by people who often, not without reason, take a jaundiced view of most clinical programs. They respect "the doctors," but they want them to mind their own business. They are concerned with the functioning of the hospital and although they welcome "good" patient labor, they do not think it their province to turn poor workers into good ones. It is up to the professionals to take care of that. They resent criticism from the professionals about the way maintenance runs, since they would not openly criticize the way "doctors" do things. Rehabilitation counselors coming around to make sure working patients were having a "therapeutic experience" were often seen as just troublemakers.

Considerable effort was made to try to allay some of the anxieties that arose with the maintenance people. For example, departments that were worried that paid work programs, as well as census reduction, would make fewer patients available for assistance were told that their amount of work would also decrease as patients were restored to the community. Where the loss of patient labor was greater than the alleviation of the work load through census reduction, we tried, and in some cases were successful, to increase the amount of regular staff help in a given area, such as the dietary department.

The PROP development was also not without its frictions and clashes. Some very prickly issues were specifically connected with linking state and private operations. At one point, a state official launched an investigation suggesting that the PROP businessmen were taking advantage of the state hospital situation by employing cheap labor and by using rent-free state facilities to reduce their overhead. Although it was true that patients were being paid below the national minimum wage, it was also true that the patients were trainees, and often very incapacitated ones, from whom less than perfect work was the rule. It was almost absurd to accuse any of the businessmen of making a personal profit. Businesses that gave contracts to PROP usually paid as much or more—in dollars and time—to PROP than they would if the job had been done elsewhere. The men did this for philanthropic reasons or as a favor to their fellow businessmen, who considered PROP their "hobby."

We might mention parenthetically that a state-hospital super-intendent would never even get started on a program involving private industry if he were to brood about possible legalistic attacks on the enterprise, such as the one in fact made by the state official on PROP. If he is sure of his own motivations and the motivations of those associated with him, he can rely on the fact that usually the truth will prevail and that one must simply be prepared to ride out the flak of sensation seekers.

We might also mention in this connection that whatever admin-istrative complications were created by the linkage of public and private organizations were more than offset by administrative gains. As an illustration, prior to PROP, the state hospital could not receive money from a state agency especially assigned to the task of rehabilitation. As a matter of fact, no state agency could directly give money to any other state agency. The establishment of PROP provided a private but nonprofit organization through which monies for rehabilitation could flow to the hospital.

However, precisely because the PROP businessmen were volunteers, and not enmeshed in the day-to-day complexities of a state institution, they had difficulty adjusting to many of the obstacles that impeded their work and dampened their enthusiasm. Not only was there the aforementioned financial issue with the state, but there were also many smaller problems that in their cumulative impact became irritating and discouraging. The hospital bureaucracy, for example, would often "forget" to meet PROP's everyday needs. One businessman complained angrily that he could not get the hospital clean-up crew to pick up the trash in back of the workshop. Several men, accustomed to being the bosses in their own small businesses, were uncomfortable not only with the bureaucratic rigidity but also with the protracted discussions, the many meetings, and the multicommittee structure of the total rehabilitation service.

Thus, it should be stressed that maintaining a complex operation like PROP is very difficult. The original enthusiasm for such a venture can easily flag in the face of the kind of obstacles just discussed, and such discouragement must be countered by repeated evidence of interest and concern on the part of administration. Both the superintendent and the assistant superintendent went to great lengths to show the PROP businessmen how much their contribution mattered to the hospital and them personally.

Work Therapy in Total Rehabilitation

It became clear over time that the work therapy program had precipitated a greater philosophic change for the hospital than had been anticipated at its inception. In terms of institutional impact, it was not merely a question of staff encouraging the vocational development of patients, of a line employee supervising a patient's work, or of a state institution cooperating with private enterprise. Rather, work therapy came to be recognized as but one aspect of the *total* rehabilitation of the chronic patient. As it eventually turned out, to be allowed to work, patients had first to meet certain criteria in dress and deportment. A great deal of learning was necessary before many could meet the standards of a sheltered workshop, and a much higher level of functioning was necessary before they could reenter the community.

The chronic patient needed confidence, a lowering of his anxiety level, and a lessening of his fear. He also needed to learn many social skills which most of us take for granted by the time we reach adulthood. Above all, he needed to feel that he could catch up on the lost years during which life had got ahead of him; he needed to overcome the defeatism, the feeling of its being "too late," which is so engrained in chronic patients.

To meet these needs, emphasis was placed on improving the social functioning of these patients. In one building, they were successfully encouraged to participate in activities that would prepare them for both work and life outside the hospital. They were taught proper grooming, the basic social amenities, and the practicalities of how to dial a telephone, use a bus, or shop in a supermarket.

This push on chronic patients toward their greater involvement in social and community life, as well as in work therapy, required constant pressure from staff. It became increasingly common for the step-system approach, a behavioral model of therapy, to be practiced in the various hospital units. In this approach, not only money but also many nonfinancial incentives for work were part of the overall reward system. For example, to gain ground privileges, the patient had to be able to dress himself and to participate in ward chores. Such a policy was not in contradiction to our open-door philosophy; it only meant that patients had to earn the right to outside privileges. If they were confined to the wards, it was not because they were, in most cases, considered dangerous, but because staff wished to exert pressure towards productivity and discourage apathy and aimless drifting.

This stress on patients earning rewards of all kinds for "correct" behavior led to many staff arguments. (It is still far from being a generally shared point of view at the hospital.) Some felt that patients had often been pushed into psychosis by family demands and expectations that they could not fulfill. The anxieties engendered, the loss of esteem, and the depressive feelings generated by failure to perform adequately in the eyes of their significant parent figures had often contributed to a downhill course. Setting up new expectations through a reward–no-reward system would put stress on the patient in exactly those areas in which he was vulnerable. However, the proponents of a reward system made the point that in the family system, failure to live up to expectations was met with rejection, ridicule, and emotional deprivations, a situation that was antithetic to the hospital's approach.

Others argued that the patient has the right to roam the grounds or have visitors regardless of whether he meets one or another social requirement. But it is our conviction that for most patients, a laissez-faire policy accomplishes little. Once again, we would emphasize the antitherapeutic significance of the implicit bargain so frequently struck up between patients, chronic and acute, and staff. If the patients do not get in staff's hair by aggressive and grossly antisocial behavior, staff will leave them alone and not urge them to do anything they do not want to do. This bargain helps avoid the many unpleasant scenes that inevitably occur when ward personnel place real expectations on patients.

But the price paid just to avoid scenes is high. Without expectations patients often sit apathetically or wander around aimlessly, trying to fill an empty day with empty diversions. Most of them *are* capable of doing something useful and *would* benefit from meeting a definite expectation. But they will not move unless staff expect them to and are prepared to pay the price of the patients' initial anger and resentment over having their static, passive equilibrium disturbed.

Some permissively oriented staff members believed that emphasis on total rehabilitation creates a concentration camp atmosphere, full of "rewards" and "punishments" demeaning to the patient's autonomy. We are not arguing for a slave-labor operation or for the use of a cattle prod to get the patient to wash his face or comb his hair. Rather, we are suggesting that forceful concern about a patient wasting his life in idleness can make him feel that somebody cares about his existence. We are further suggesting that once the patient gains some self-esteem through purposeful activity, he will begin to value his own existence.

The administrator consistently had to support those physicians, nurses, and work therapists who practiced this philosophy in the face of counterarguments and resistances. He tried to increase the resources, prestige, and power of such persons in their efforts to get patients moving. Eventually this behavioral approach to total rehabilitation gained legitimacy in the hospital and became a full-fledged ideology of patient care along with other treatment modalities.

REFERENCES

1. Melvin Cohen, "Work as a Therapeutic Tool in the State Mental Hospital," *Mental Hygiene* 49, no. 3 (July 1965): 358–63.

2. T. Schoenfeld, unpublished data on PROP, 1965.

CHAPTER 7

Volunteers

A recurrent theme in this book has been the grievous discrepancy between the almost limitless needs of the mentally ill and the limited resources a state hospital can command to meet them. One significant way this crucial gap can be bridged is by the intelligent recruitment and assignment of volunteers, or, in a larger sense, by citizen participation.

It is our conviction that volunteers represent the latent resource which, uncovered and fully and appropriately utilized, can make the difference between a marginal existence and an acceptable life for the hospitalized. Even in states most enlightened in their care of the emotionally ill patients, the large mental hospital and indeed almost all psychiatric facilities suffer from severe shortages in staff and materiel.

Not only do volunteers represent the potential for significant quantitative increase in manpower, but they also provide a qualitative impact that is distinctly different from that of professional staff. Patients quickly sense or recognize that volunteers work at the hospital solely because of personal interest and a desire to be helpful rather than because they are pursuing a career. Their very lack of professionalism means that patients can have some relatively spontaneous and natural associations with "normal" people without being inhibited by the provisos that some professionals, particularly anxious beginners, bring to their relationships with patients. We do not wish to imply that these relationships are more effective than those undertaken by professional staff, but that their quality is different and this difference seems to be a positive one, especially for chronic patients with whom most volunteers work.

It has sometimes been argued that since most large mental hospitals are reducing their inpatient census, there should be less need of additional personnel, volunteers or otherwise. This argument is fallacious; discharged patients badly need follow-up care if they are to remain out of the hospital, thus continuing their demand on staff time and efforts, which are already being taxed by multiplying numbers of outpatient admissions. Moreover, most mental health institutions, and particularly those in urban areas, have become increasingly involved in a whole network of community socioemotional problems, such as drug addiction, juvenile delinquency, and even learning problems. These community concerns put even more strain on the energies of continually undermanned and overworked staff.

One inpatient problem especially dramatizes the need for volunteer help. With the return of many patients to the community, the population remaining in the hospital is composed largely of chronic, "burnt-out" emotional casualties who often incur in staff a feeling of defeatism. Furthermore, the work rehabilitation project notwithstanding, most new, imaginative programs are directed toward acute patients, and staff not unnaturally are drawn toward what they believe is more intellectually stimulating and rewarding work, where positive gains are often seen within a circumscribed period of time. In this climate there is a particular need for enthusiastic, motivated volunteers with a special interest in working with those to whom destiny has given such a poor hand of cards to play.

The chronic shortages of most public institutions become acute in a period when tax monies for social needs are in scarce supply, an impasse that confronts us at the time of writing. No longer can staff automatically think in terms of new state or federally financed programs to complete unfinished tasks or to start new projects. If a public institution wishes to continue to improve its treatment programs, it must utilize volunteers to help man its services far more than it had in the past.

Thus, especially in periods of governmental belt-tightening we would do well to give the ordinary citizen a role in the structure of social and health services and the kind of support that will fire his interest and imagination. In so doing, we have an opportunity to counteract the trend toward the depersonalization of large professional bureaucracies, which so isolate and estrange the lay citizen. Such alienation is particularly detrimental to community mental health programs, which depend upon engagement from the people themselves and not just from the agencies presumably representing them. More of our energies must be devoted to involving the lay public in the overwhelming mental health problems confronting us in the hospital, the clinic, and the community at large.

Fortunately, the psychiatric profession's increasing awareness of the need for volunteers resonates with major themes in the larger culture. Volunteering has always played an important part in American life, stemming back to colonial times, and its salience and scope had markedly increased during the socially conscious and fermenting 1960s.

The mental health domain has a singularly attractive potential for recruiting diverse kinds of volunteers.[1] Students interested in learning about themselves, as well as about the dynamics of mental illness, and in helping a deprived, disfranchised group can find, and often have found, the mental hospital the answer to meet their needs for both relevant education and community service. Older individuals, with shorter working hours than ever in history, can find that helping the mentally ill is one way of giving satisfaction and meaning to their leisure time. Citizens living in the community the hospital serves have a direct stake in participating in mental health activities that may affect some member of their family or their friends. Moreover, increasing information about the psychology of man, communicated to the public by mass media, has made a quite widespread population realize that helping others is one way of helping themselves.

The reader may well ask why we speak of citizen participation as the *latent* resource if the desire to volunteer is so strong and the need for volunteers so great. The reasons are manifold; here, we will allude only to the more important ones.

The same factors that lead to underutilization of nonmedical personnel within the hospital apply with double force to prevent the full development of the volunteer's role. Too often, his participation is limited to only such good-Samaritan functions as arranging Christmas parties for patients or raising funds for hospital improvement. To many professional staff, the very definition of mental illness as a disease entity has implied that only highly trained staff can perform important tasks with patients. Perhaps the shaky state of psychiatry as a science has made us anxious and defensive about the full utilization of volunteers lest they reveal just how much untrained people can do. Moreover, there still remains a tacit agreement among some members of our society that the government alone should assume responsibility for our medically indigent population and should provide adequate staff to meet their needs.

Nonetheless, the current trend is toward inviting citizen participation and many institutions now have active volunteer programs. In the next section we shall describe various volunteer groups at Boston State, in terms of their history, interests, and functions.

Volunteer Groups

For purposes of exposition, we have divided the different groups under four major rubrics—traditional volunteers, student volunteers, nonstudent case aides, and government-appointed volunteers. The many and sometimes taxing administrative problems in dealing with volunteers will be considered after we conclude our descriptive survey.

Traditional Volunteers

For many years individual citizens, benevolent and steeped in the tradition of volunteerism, have dedicated themselves to visiting the lonely and forgotten in the back wards of mental hospitals. They have brought food, clothing, and even money to patients toward whom they felt sympathetic.

Or such generous people have functioned in similar ways as part of an organization. The Friends of the Hospital, for example, a group of about five hundred women who live in the area Boston State serves, have made extraordinary contributions in personal services, money, physical-plant improvement, and legislative activities. Other civic, labor, and veterans' organizations (about seventy-five to one hundred in all) have arranged for special holiday parties for patients and contributed goods and services to the hospital.

It has become somewhat fashionable to minimize the importance of this kind of volunteering. Undoubtedly, some of what these volunteers do has a trace of the old-time Lady Bountiful, who distributed her charity to the dispossessed and the downtrodden, but almost always at arm's length. However, given the appalling material deprivation of a state hospital, an administrator errs badly if he slights or underestimates the worth of traditional volunteers. Their very absence of deep psychological interest in patients makes them more inclined to become involved in fund-raising, building renovation, recreational events, parties, and dances—practical projects that enhance the living conditions of the patients and lift the morale of the hospital generally. Although they lack the zeal for reform that characterizes the younger volunteers, they can be depended upon to respond when they are called.

A further advantage not to be overlooked is that most of the traditional volunteers live in the immediate hospital area, putting them in an excellent position to be a transitional link for patients returning to the community. They know who would be receptive to employing a former patient, where he would be welcome as a roomer, and where he can get a helping hand.

Student Volunteers

If the groups just described represent the prototype of volunteering of the past, the student movement represents a new spirit that is spreading among volunteers of all ages.

The modern history of the student volunteer effort in state hospitals was started by Harvard and Radcliffe undergraduates in 1954 with a burst of excitement and an unstinted enthusiasm for work with the mentally ill.[2] The revolutionary passion that characterized the college campus of the 1930s had been quieted considerably by the McCarthy investigation of the early 1950s, as well as by a host of other social factors that contributed to the "silent generation" of college students during that period. However, a good deal of reform spirit, restive below the surface, was waiting to be directed into appropriate channels. The impact of the Freudian psychological revolution on the young makes it logical in retrospect that their reform spirit was first directed toward the mental hospital rather than toward such later concerns as the civil rights issues of the South and the ghetto problems of the North.

We have mentioned earlier in this text the pivotal role of single individuals in initiating large organizational changes; the student volunteer movement also had its charismatic leader. In 1954, an inspired sophomore at Harvard, having seen in the previous year the poverty and deprivation of the mental hospital, opened the way for the release of student energies. He led some five hundred undergraduates on a tour through the dark corridors of state institutions, laid the responsibility for action on their shoulders, and held up to them the vision of patient rehabilitation and discharge that could be directly attributed to their personal efforts.

Before school got under way that fall, a recruiting rally was held at which the needs of the hospital were dramatically highlighted by staff representatives and student leaders. Hundreds signed up for work on the wards as quasi-recreational and occupational therapists. Initially, the students directed their efforts toward working with groups of patients—having discussions, organizing ward activities and outside excursions, teaching games, and so on.

From this beginning, the students evolved two very special programs. The first was a case-aide venture which permitted them to establish, with supervision, close, continued, one-to-one relationships with patients. Here, as in their group activities, they were most often challenged by chronic patients with whom regular staff had failed. The relationships they developed varied widely, depending on the needs of the patients and the interests of the students. For example, one Harvard undergraduate developed a close association with a middle-aged schizophrenic woman who had been hospitalized for thirty years. The student, who was in analysis himself, was supported and supervised in this venture by a staff physician. Over a period of two years, the patient's speech changed from incomprehensible mutterings to coherent communication. Slowly, she began to take an interest in the world around her and started the tortuous climb to recovery. Other students, working with better functioning patients, directed themselves from the start to such issues as work therapy and return to community living. Indeed, getting patients out of the hospital was a strong leitmotif for many of these young volunteers.

The lack of adequate transitional facilities for former patients who were not quite ready to go it alone led some student volunteers to create a second major innovation—a halfway house where patients and students lived together. This facility, which was several miles from the hospital, was run largely by the students themselves, with professionals serving only as consultants.

It should not be thought that these eager young students were welcomed with open arms when they first offered their services. On the contrary, they had to *push* their way in because staff met their first efforts with much anxiety, skepticism, and resistance. But possessing rebellious spirits and evangelical fervor, they showed that they could not only survive, but also improve the physical and social environment, make direct and beneficial contacts with chronic patients, and establish true innovations. As a result, the hospital experienced what it had never known before: a mass influx of enthusiastic young people, intelligent, motivated, bent on improvement, and drawn to the worst wards, challenged by patients who had been labeled hopeless.

By and large, the students administered their own programs, requesting help only when absolutely necessary. Although they wanted to learn from professional staff, they did not want to be controlled by them. In a self-sustaining way, they continued to recruit many new colleagues each year from the schools in the Boston area.

We may say a few words about another, most interesting volunteer status, largely but not entirely composed of students, modeled on the Peace Corps. Some financial support is given to these semivolunteers, sufficient to prevent them from dipping too deeply into their own pockets, yet not enough to diminish the altruistic component of volunteering. The group includes VISTA volunteers, some of whose members serve in mental health programs. Indeed, Boston State was the first facility to obtain VISTAs for mental hospital work. Others came to the hospital through a special statefinanced program, the Commonwealth Service Corps, and through various individual arrangements whereby the hospital provided some kind of material support, usually board and room and a below-minimum hourly wage. Unlike the student volunteer program per se, this kind of volunteering permits students and others to spend substantial blocks of time at the hospital, either during a dropout year from college or during a summer vacation. Moreover, it opens up all kinds of possibilities for staffing, even on a temporary basis, hard-to-fill positions, such as attendants for the evening shift, with enthusiastic young men and women.

Nonstudent Case Aides

In 1963, Boston State received a small grant from a private foundation to demonstrate that intelligent and motivated older volunteers could, with proper supervision, establish therapeutic relationships with chronically ill patients.[3]

The volunteers' responding to recruitment efforts consisted largely, as is the case with most groups interested in community affairs, of well-to-do, college-educated, middle-aged men and women. The kinds of relationships they made with patients resembled those of the student volunteers: partly therapeutic, partly educational, and partly supportive, a mixture that brought positive gains to many long-term cases.

A distinctive feature of the case-aide program was that it

recruited a group of people who could make a *sustained* commitment relatively uninterrupted by school vacations, study and exam periods, or sudden shifts in interest. Like traditional volunteers, case aides accepted assignments more readily than students and were more tolerant of the idiosyncracies of staff.

Indirectly, the case-aide program helped provide current knowledge about mental health to a group of citizens who could utilize that information well in their community roles. Because of their hospital experience, they could be stimulated to join their local mental health association or to play a more active role in diverse kinds of city-wide citizen organizations that concerned themselves with community problems of all kinds.

Another distinctive feature of the program was its careful administrative structure. Whereas students often preferred to work largely on their own, the older group, being more hesitant, needed and received close, sustained support. This help was given by a group of experienced social workers who, like most of the case aides, were usually married women with families. Use of a group method of supervision permitted just a few part-time social workers to train more than one hundred case aides, thereby vastly expanding direct service to patients with a minimum of additional professional expense. Moreover, another valuable administrative policy was the training of talented and experienced case aides to serve as supervisors of new case aides.

We believe this use of volunteers as staff contains an important administrative principle. In many new programs of this kind, there is a tendency to remain fast in the original mode of functioning, for example, one social-work supervisor for every eight volunteers. Thus, expansion is frequently blocked by the limitations of professional manpower. Making capable volunteers themselves teachers of volunteers allows the possibility for continuing expansion of the program without depending on increased funds.

Government-appointed or Statutory Volunteers

The different volunteer groups just described have in common a concern with individual patients or with ward or service projects.

None is involved with planning for the hospital's direction as a whole or with the overall relationships between the hospital and its community. We turn now to two statutory groups—the hospital board of trustees and the area boards—which do have these generalized functions as specific parts of their governmental mandate.

At Boston State, as at other institutions of the Massachusetts Department of Mental Health, the board of trustees is appointed by the governor, and each member of the seven-citizen board serves for a period of seven years. Trustees are enjoined to inspect hospital facilities, examine records, advise on policy and appointments, and function as a nonprofit corporation receiving funds, bequests, grants, and donations of land to be disposed of as they wish. Since the board is most often made up of prominent citizens, they usually have access to important sources of influence, such as labor organizations, legislators, and professional groups.

In addition to their collective functions, individual members of the board of trustees can perform very important volunteer roles in part because their interest is stimulated directly by the superintendent's urging and in part because their role carries more official weight than that of the usual volunteer. At Boston State, during our tenure, one former trustee became involved in the PROP program; another was instrumental in planning for a night hospital. Several trustees made the condition of various hospital buildings their concern, a watchdog function the board was well designed to fill. Since trustees are volunteers who by decree must report directly to the governor, their criticisms had to be carefully attended to.

In terms of representing the community the hospital serves, however, the board works under two distinct disadvantages: members are appointed by the governor, with little or no say from the community itself, and there is no stipulation that they must reside or work in the hospital catchment area.

The regional plan mentioned in the chapter on unitization highlighted the need for more direct and immediate citizen participation at a statutory level. This plan, the reader will recall, involved Boston State's becoming a community mental health center for a catchment area of two hundred thousand people. The hospital's new overall psychiatric responsibility for a discrete geographic area raised with particular cogency the question of citizen involvement from the community the hospital served. To meet this need, the regional plan, implemented by law in 1966, called for governmentally identified and created area boards. This new law directed the department of mental health to establish citizen boards for each of its thirty-seven mental health service areas and stipulated that the area boards should consist of twenty-one members "who shall be appointed by the Commissioner. Two-thirds of the members shall live within the area for which they are appointed and the remaining members shall either live or work within said area. . . ."

The particular issues that developed between Boston State and its area board are outside the scope of this volume. However, more general problems concerning the relationship between a hospital and a statutory citizen group, whether hospital trustees or an area board, will be discussed at the end of the next section.

Administrative Issues

A critical issue common to all volunteer efforts is proper supervision and assignment of tasks. All too often good volunteers either leave or perform inadequately because they are not given the right task or because they get insufficient assistance when performing even a well-placed assignment. The burden of supervision is often left to only one person—the paid director of volunteers—with few staff members sharing any of this responsibility. In a hospital with more than a handful of volunteers, such an arrangement is patently inadequate.

Student volunteers often use their own pooled funds to pay for professional guidance, which does help take up some of the supervisory slack. However, these consultants often concern themselves with the student-patient relationship rather than with the student-hospital collaboration. This leaves a large administrative gap in terms of the enormous amount of coordinating that has to be done

between the volunteers and the hospital, such as mediating difficulties that arise between volunteers and ward staff or helping
worthwhile volunteers obtain extra resources to develop special
programs. Such coordinating functions can only be handled by
persons who understand the complexities of the volunteer's role
and who can give the time required for proper supervision.

The preceding does not necessarily mean that the director of
volunteers' staff must consist entirely of professional persons. As
pointed out in the case aide program, some talented volunteers
with a special commitment to working with the emotionally ill
can themselves become supervisors of new and inexperienced
recruits. We found that over time these case aides developed
skills not only in supervising the novice volunteer in his clinical
work, but also acquired sufficient familiarity with the hospital
to guide the new persons through the complex mazes of its social
system.

The use of volunteers as supervisors is important both because
of the additional training manpower it provides without cost and
because it helps work against another common administrative
problem in dealing with volunteers—professionalism. If volunteers
are forced into a Procrustean bed of staff habits and attitudes in
dealing with patients, it can dampen their enthusiasm and rob
them of their spontaneity, two assets that make volunteers so
invaluable in working with the chronically ill.

Some administrators favor a quite controlled volunteer program
right from the start, with very careful interviews and tests to
determine a volunteer's fitness to work with the mentally ill on the
basis of his having the "right motivation," the "right personality
type," and other such shibboleths. In our experience, such a view
is unrealistic, if not almost self-defeating. With the incalculable
need of the mentally ill for care and attention and with the
enormous choice of assignment possible in our present system,
we believe it is folly to exclude anyone on some vague basis of
his not being the "right kind of person." Barring flagrant misfits,
it is often very difficult to predict whether a volunteer will excel
in his efforts or whether he will fail. The talents of volunteers who

would have been screened out initially on the basis of dogmatic criteria can be creatively utilized by providing the proper kind of activity, a degree of supervision, and administrative flexibility. True, there will always be those who do not work out. But we believe it best for them to screen themselves out over time—and it usually does not take a great deal of time—rather than risk the chance of arbitrarily refusing a borderline candidate who might have turned out to be a great asset to the program.

Neither is there complete agreement about indoctrination. Some programs go to great lengths to see that the volunteer is properly indoctrinated; others let him plunge right in and learn from experience. Since each individual learns in his own way and it is difficult to ascertain the impact of scheduled instruction, there cannot be one pat formula that will apply to all volunteers. Rather, the significant factor is whether the volunteer is given the proper opportunities. These include the opportunity for volunteer and supervisor together to become committed to a mutual task; to discuss in depth the meaning of the patient's behavior within the context of the treatment system and the significance to the patient's welfare of the technique and style of intervention practiced by the individual volunteer; to share pressing concerns, anxieties, and frustrations; and to integrate experience and thus add to one's knowledge.

The tensions and frustrations that inevitably arise from working with the mentally ill will affect the volunteer just as they do other staff members. (We use the word *other* advisedly; volunteers should always be considered as part of staff.) The volunteer often needs time and he certainly needs help in assimilating his experiences. Furthermore, unresponsive chronic patients leave the volunteer with a sense of failure and discouragement; the skilled supervisor will try to help him over these periods of low morale. Again, like other staff members, the volunteer should have open to him opportunities for continuous in-service training to make him feel part of the therapeutic organization and to improve his effectiveness and increase his job satisfaction.

Some of the subtleties involved in furnishing the right kind of supervision can best be illustrated by discussing a specific group of volunteers, the students. Here, having some understanding of the motives for volunteering is particularly helpful in designing a system of supervision. Students often come to the hospital with a strong desire to learn about mental illness and about their own emotional conflicts. Many are also contemplating careers in psychiatry and wish to have the opportunity to see if mature professionals in this field are the kinds of persons they wish to emulate. Both these motives lead students to want to have contact with trained persons and to be supervised by them.

At the same time, students have a compelling need to protest and rebel against the adult world that has fashioned such a degrading life for its emotional casualties, against the rigidities of an institutional system that resists change and new ideas, against prisonlike restraint, against boredom and monotony, and against the finality of the shattering prognosis of "hopeless," so often given to chronic mental patients. Students are also in a stage in their life cycle when they have a strong need for autonomy, a need which expresses itself in the hospital setting as a desire for freedom and sanction to select their own patients and to work with them in any constructive way they wish.

The supervisory knack lies in providing enough guidance to meet the learning needs of the students, but eschewing the kind of control they feel threatens their idealism, autonomy, and creativity. Students are often angered by tutors who offer psychological reasons for their rebelliousness or rescue fantasies about patients without empathizing with their genuine, and quite rational, moral indignation over much that goes on at a state hospital. Also, they are very impatient with supervisors who arbitrarily dismiss avant-garde psychiatric concepts and techniques, often so appealing to young people. They rightly sense that some professionals do this because of their own defensiveness, dogmatism, and need to justify the psychiatric status quo.

If an administrator really appreciates the kinds of contributions student volunteers can make and the desperate need of a mental hospital for their ingenuity and vitality, he will make it a point to cultivate those professionals who can guide students without inhibiting them, a kind of supervisory talent too little explored or defined. For example, a good supervisor of psychiatric residents is not necessarily a good supervisor of college students. So far, it is the good supervisor of professionals who has been most rewarded in many hospital systems, whereas talent with volunteers is taken as an epiphenomenon—nice, but not indispensable.

The intrusive evangelism of student volunteers can be threatening not only to professional supervisors, but to the entire hospital staff as well, from the attendant to the top administrator. It takes considerable self-security and tolerance on the part of the administrator to create the kind of liberal atmosphere within which students can experiment in a variety of ways, albeit with sufficient control to prevent truly destructive excesses. Some administrators live in dread that the students will commit some youthful folly that will eventuate in a newspaper scandal. If the administrator exerts oppressive controls to preclude the possibility of even a minor indiscretion, he will find few student recruits for his hospital.

Even if supervisory staff and top administration are receptive to student volunteers, there may still be considerable resistance to them among lower-level personnel. We have found that attendants, particularly, often treated students like ubiquitous visitors —to be tolerated, but only with the utmost caution. They feared a disruption of routine and an increase in work, but most of all they were afraid they would be pushed out of their jobs. They generally resented these young outsiders, who were often of a higher social class and better educated than they. They also felt, and not without cause, that the students did not appreciate the day-to-day arduous tasks they were performing in handling intractable patients or in encouraging apathetic ones. The antipathy was not necessarily limited to personnel on the wards where the students worked, but sometimes reached into higher echelons, where it was manifested by suspiciousness, fear of criticism, and concern about possible harm to patients.

One way of handling this problem was to include ward personnel in the initial planning of student activities in their particular area. When feasible, students were asked to help ward workers directly with those patients the employees considered the most difficult to manage. Another kind of solution was to bypass the hospital structure as much as possible by affording students the opportunity to run their own show, pretty much apart from hospital regulations. This is the way they functioned in the half-way house, where professionals served only as consultants, and the day-to-day operation was run entirely by students. This kind of arrangement can unleash students' energies to a very high pitch without the impediment of daily arguments with ward staff. It has the disadvantage, however, of withdrawing from the hospital system itself the much-needed creative drive and earnestness of dedicated young people.

Much of what we have written regarding administrative tasks with student volunteers applies to semivolunteers, with a few additional problems. Attracting semivolunteers attached to VISTA, OEO-funded projects, and college work-study programs requires considerable alertness on the part of the administrator. He must know what programs are current and must be energetic in demonstrating the feasibility and desirability of the hospital for volunteers. Sometimes, when the institution must supply a modest amount of matching money, he must exert considerable ingenuity to find some unallocated funds. It is likely he will run into considerable red tape in an effort to provide the simplest prerequisites, such as room and board for eligible persons who are eager to volunteer their services but who need some minimum sustenance. Only if the administrator truly recognizes the value of such volunteers will he go to all the trouble necessary to get them installed. And only if the semivolunteers fit into some rational design and get the proper supervision, will his efforts be worth their while.

We mentioned earlier that semivolunteers are often in a position to take on major assignments over an extended period of time, tasks they are prepared to perform not only because of their altruistic desire to be of service but also because of the educational opportunities offered them at a state hospital. Administratively, their utilization can raise serious problems with the hospital labor union who objects to anyone, semivolunteers or not, working for substandard wages. The problem becomes particularly acute if the administrator divides up one regular, but unfilled position, to give some maintenance income to several semivolunteers. To some extent, he can quiet the union on this issue by pointing out that prior to the employment of the students, the position could not be filled, so that no one is being deprived of a job.

Some administrative differences in dealing with older volunteers emerge as early as the time of recruitment. Whereas word spreads quickly in the student world about the volunteering possibilities at a given institution, deliberate and well-planned efforts have to be made to attract nonstudent volunteers. For example, it took considerable publicity of all kinds in all parts of Boston to recruit a sufficient number of volunteers to start the case aide program and then to help it grow.

In terms of placement and supervision, nonstudent groups often wish more structured tasks than students, but are more compliant about fitting into hospital expectations. Some, particularly case aides, also want close relationships with patients, but seek more specific supervision than students often do. It is wise, administratively, to insure that they obtain such supervision from the start in a regular, organized fashion.

Other nonstudent volunteers definitely do not wish to get too close to patients; their efforts should be directed in a way that is congruent with their desire to be helpful, even though removed. The administrator must search for the staff person or persons who appreciate these volunteers and want to help them organize social activities, renovate buildings, and the like.

In this context, the administrator's problem with staff is not so much resistance to this group of volunteers, since they do not intrude in staff's bailiwick. Rather, it is that staff, principally psychotherapy-oriented professionals, are often indifferent to, or undervalue, the worth of this kind of effort. The administrator is also less likely to hear about the dissatisfaction of older volunteers since they are not so prone to rush in with their complaints. Rather, they are more likely to suffer silently and in time quietly depart.

A sensitive director of volunteers can alleviate some of these difficulties by a proper diagnosis of which staff members work best with which volunteers, rather than simply applying an automatic yardstick of so many volunteers to so many staff members. In our experience, older staff members frequently do better with more traditionally oriented volunteers, whereas younger professionals are more receptive to students. Obvious as this may seem, it still takes some acuity, determination, and schedule-shifting to match certain volunteers with certain staff. We might also mention in this connection that given the grave shortages of ward staff, there is often a tendency to diffuse the volunteers throughout the hospital. However, if volunteers are not in a position to get support from each other, they often feel bewildered and isolated. In times of volunteer shortages, it is more prudent to concentrate the volunteers on a given service, even at the expense of temporary neglect of other facilities. The more successful experiences of volunteers who have obtained support from each other will enhance the overall recruitment effort through their word-of-mouth publicity.

In dealing with volunteers of all kinds, the administrator, or his deputies, must perform many seemingly routine but nonetheless vitally important tasks. Some have to do with the volunteers' work with patients, usually help from the "main office" in negotiating a problem they encountered on a particular ward. Or they may want help from the administrator himself in getting outside funds to finance a special project, such as a summer camp. In other instances, the help they seek may be personal: a letter of recommendation or temporary summer employment as a paid staff member.

In addition to personal favors, older volunteers often seek and should be rewarded with some tangible recognition of their work —service pins, appointments to hospital committees, newspaper publicity, and the like. We may add, parenthetically, that unlike voluntary hospitals most state institutions have neglected the judicious use of such concrete awards in running their volunteer programs. It is rare to see even a ward, let alone a special building, named after a lay citizen who has rendered distinguished service to the hospital.

Like students, older volunteers also have their more personal reasons for volunteering, and these are frequently connected with their interest in a mentally ill relative or friend. They often have a strong desire to talk about their near one's condition and their own feelings of guilt about it. A sensitive supervisor can be most helpful to them within the framework of volunteering rather than in the more usual framework of their consulting someone directly involved with the case.

Indeed, we may mention here that it is often the sense of frustration that relatives of patients feel about the hospital and the frustration staff feels about relatives that prevent the full mobilization of a very natural volunteer group—those who have seen the ravages of mental illness at close quarters. Relatives and friends have a private reason for wanting to improve the hospital and they know firsthand many of its deficiencies. However, staff are often reluctant to hear once again the relatives' poignant pleas or their criticism of this or that aspect of a program that concerns their near ones. Intelligent handling of such volunteers includes a readiness to listen to some of their immediate concerns as well as a capacity to channel the interest of those persons into efforts that will benefit many patients, not just those they are directly concerned with.

If the administrator is responsive to the different motives, needs, and rewards for all kinds of volunteers, he creates the kind of ambiance in which volunteers flourish. This does not mean that he must constantly lean backward to show his gratitude for their service. Both staff and administrator must constantly keep in mind that volunteers are not personally helping *them*, but are helping the patients or the community.

An unsolved administrative problem in working with volunteers of all kinds is finding the way to utilize them most effectively at the time they are most needed—the evening shift (from three to eleven). Many hospitals virtually close down at this time, just when patients most often need individual attention, as well as some group activity. Students and older volunteers who work during the day are often particularly keen to involve themselves at the hospital during precisely those hours when they are most needed. But it is during these hours that they are least likely to get proper supervision, since regular staff have gone home. Moreover, there tends to be a drifting of more custodial-minded supervisory personnel toward the evening and night shifts because during these quiet hours they are less likely to be bothered by either upper-level staff or students. Volunteers and custodial-minded personnel make a bad combination; student volunteers have complained that when they came in the evening they sometimes found that the ward had been locked to them or that the patients had been deliberately put to bed early, usually for some fictitious reason. Personnel in turn have complained about one or another indiscretion on the part of the students which in turn led them to restrict their activities. The mediating hand of skilled professionals, interested in the students but cognizant of the problems posed by ward personnel, is absent during the evening hours, just when it is most needed.

We might mention one current problem in recruiting volunteers that applies to most women, young and middle-aged alike. The location of Boston State in an urban area has in the past been an outstanding advantage for attracting volunteers. However, with the rising concern about violence in the inner city, most women are loathe to travel after dark. On a short-term basis, certain administrative steps can be taken to allay this fear, for example, by using busses to transport volunteers. From a more long-term perspective, the question of the hospital's relationship with its immediate community is again raised. Slum-ridden, disorganized communities are not only a breeding ground for mental illness, but they can also pose, in the form of violence, or the fear of it, a very real obstacle in obtaining help of any kind, let alone volunteers.

The danger is also an opportunity. Whereas students in the

early 1950s concentrated mainly on care of the mentally ill as the focus for volunteering, today the mental hospital competes for crusading volunteers with a host of other social organizations, especially those concerned with the problems of the ghetto. If the hospital can link its activities to a very wide framework that includes stress on community work in deprived areas, it will be in a far better position to attract students and others interested in the social as well as the psychological determinants of emotional illness.

The problem of recruiting volunteers in an increasingly tense urban atmosphere highlights the issue of citizen involvement with the total problems of a large mental hospital. As we have mentioned, most hospital volunteers assume relatively circumscribed tasks without concerning themselves about overall hospital issues. Lay groups who will share this responsibility with the hospital administration are sorely needed, particularly in the area of hospital-community relations. However, in working with such groups a host of dilemmas arise, mostly concerned with the proper relationship between government-appointed citizen groups and mental health professionals. In our opinion, it is more important at this point in time to raise the right questions concerning this collaboration rather than to presume any final answers.

One such key question is the issue of power. How are the prerogatives of decision-making distributed between the citizen group on one hand and the superintendent and his staff on the other? The emphasis nowadays is on increased power for the citizenry, just as it was in a different sense some time ago when a statutory group of lay citizens, the boards of trustees of state hospitals in Massachusetts, had considerable authority. Not only did they appoint the superintendent, but subordinate officers as well. Since they were not actively involved in the day-to-day operation of the hospital, their factual knowledge was insufficient to justify their ultimate power of decision regarding appointments or policy development. The granting of such authority to an outside group of citizens may have seemed justified on the grounds that they did not have the vested interest of staff, but in fact they often had their own axes to grind. Furthermore, when the board had such great control, the command of leadership became divided, with the superintendent often in a quite weak position. The subsequent harm to staff morale necessitated in the 1950s a sharp circumscription of the trustees' authority, which eventually led to their taking the more advisory position they have today.

It may be argued that the board of trustees was not the appropriate citizen body to be given such influence since most of the trustees did not live in the community the institution served and were not chosen by the community to represent it. The reader will recall that another statutory group, the area board, was established precisely to have a citizen group more representative of the community. Nevertheless, the members of the area board, like the trustees, are not directly involved in the daily functioning of the hospital. Thus, the question still remains: How much decision-making power should these groups have?

If we have stressed some of the pitfalls of excessive power in the citizens' hands, we should equally stress the pitfalls of too little power. A purely advisory role, although congenial to some people, is unlikely to make a citizen group truly effective. Such a group can easily turn into being a rubber stamp for the hospital administration or be used as another route to social climbing for members more interested in the prestige of the appointment than in the actual challenges facing the institution and its community.

The issue of power is closely linked to the issue of what kinds of citizens are appointed to the boards. Even when, as in the case of the area boards, various efforts are made to achieve widespread representation, there is a tendency for more middle-class, college-educated, professional (and lay) citizens to be appointed and to be given positions of leadership on such boards than it is for less educated and less affluent citizens to achieve this distinction. If a middle-class board has considerable power in a community housing mainly lower-class citizens, the community as a whole might be no better represented than when all power chiefly resides in the hands of hospital staff.

We have highlighted these dilemmas not to evoke a sense of

despair but to be realistic about the challenges confronting us in a conflictual, emotion-charged realm—community involvement vis-à-vis public institutions. No one can provide a detailed prescription as a panacea for all the intricacies of this issue. We will, however, suggest some thoughts on the administrative stance toward statutory groups.

We believe that in dealing with government-appointed groups of volunteers, the administrator's attitude should be as open and experimental as it is toward individual volunteers. As with individual volunteers, he will very likely find that when the issue of power becomes a crucial one, inadequacy is often the underlying problem rather than the question of who controls whom or who can outvote whom.

We found, for example, that individual volunteers can often function most effectively in an area where staff are least effective—dealing with chronic patients. Given this capacity, we granted considerable decision-making opportunities to student volunteers, even to allowing them to run their own halfway houses and the like. Abused, defensive feelings on the part of staff had to be dealt with, as did overzealous demands for instant hospital reform on the part of the students.

The same general model applies to statutory groups. Community groups, for example, are likely to know more about the key mental health issues in their neighborhood than professionals. Just as it would be a mistake for an administrator to allow lay citizens to decide whether a patient should be given electroconvulsive therapy or an antidepressant drug, so it would be equally a mistake to allow professional staff on its own to decide whether a drug addiction unit or a new center for geriatric patients should have first priority in a given community.

Even when community citizens are involved in determining whether a particular facility will be developed, they are often too little included in the actual planning. Just as local citizens often have the firsthand knowledge to determine the priorities of need in the community, so they are also in an excellent position to build a widespread community consensus for a particular project and to help coalesce clusters of creativity that can make the new program function vigorously. They can only do this if the administrator encourages them to play an active role at all stages of its development.

A large part of the administrator's task with statutory groups lies in involving them in areas where their own skills and experiences can come fully into play. It also lies in helping his own staff learn how to work collaboratively with such groups so that staff can serve as catalysts, coordinators, and sources of particular kinds of expertise. When lay citizens and professionals are drawn together in a common interest, when each has particular skills to contribute toward achieving a common goal, cries of "more power" or "look at what the amateurs are doing" are less likely to be heard.

The administrator and his staff can make good use of their clinical skills in dealing with statutory groups, especially if they do so discreetly. With their psychiatric acumen, they can recognize the potential troublemaker, whether he be a disgruntled militant demanding instant action or a successful executive who believes that because he has operated his business well he should also be in charge of the hospital or its community programs.

The administrator's challenge here is not to let his enthusiasm for volunteers and their potential be dampened by awareness of their limitations. No matter who the volunteers are, almost all have difficulty comprehending the subtleties and complexities of mental illness. They also are frequently unaware of their own biases and neurotic trends as they interfere with the perception of problems. The idealism which in part led them to volunteer in the first place may also be accompanied by an impatience that blinds them to the difficulties attendant to social change, to the rights of dissenters, and to the time needed to build a consensus necessary to institute a new program.

We would err if we ended this chapter by stressing the administrative problems with statutory groups, or, for that matter, with volunteers in general. Rather, we would prefer to close by reiterating that the administrative challenge to uncover the hidden resources of community participation is perhaps one of the most important efforts confronting leadership in the human services today. Whether one focuses on direct treatment of the severely ill or on trying to alleviate the social ills that poison emotional development, one must recognize the many-sided and indispensable role of the volunteer.

In this perspective, all that has been described above is but a trifle compared to the full potential for citizen participation that exists in the population. For every group working in the hospital, there are many more in the community indirectly involved in promoting the mental health of the people. Every service organization and every political and social group dedicated to improving the nature of the city, eliminating discrimination, rebuilding slums, decreasing crime and delinquency, improving physical health, abolishing poverty, or advancing education—all serve to minimize or eliminate the many causes contributing to mental illness. Some groups operate with little conscious recognition of the important role they are playing; others clearly appreciate the effects of their activities in reducing the psychological hazards of life and in rendering aid to mental and emotional casualties.

Some may say that these diverse efforts have long gone on and could continue to function without the aid of mental health professionals. We argue that the psychiatric professions do have an important role to play with the community groups. No longer can there be any clear distinction between mental illness on the one hand and a host of social disorders on the other. We, in the mental hospital, desperately need the community's help with our specific tasks; the community desperately needs our help—help, not command—in dealing with its myriad difficulties, so many of which have a clear-cut emotional component. It is not easy, but it is crucial that the mental health administrator constantly reassess his utilization of professionals and lay citizens, that he constantly ask his staff and himself: What hospital tasks now being done by professionals could be done as well or better by volunteers? How can such volunteers be mobilized? What community groups or efforts can staff fruitfully catalyze in a way that may ameliorate or eliminate emotional disturbance so that the need for hospitalization or even outpatient treatment will be drastically reduced?

We cannot predict the answers to these questions. But we do not hesitate to prophesy that, partly because of the increased use of volunteers, the patterns of psychiatric functioning will be as different thirty years from now as they were thirty years ago.

REFERENCES

1. P. L. Ewalt, ed., *Mental Health Volunteers: The Expanding Role of the Volunteer in Hospital and Community Mental Health Services* (Springfield, Ill.: Charles C Thomas, 1966).

2. J. L. Dohan, "Development of a Student Volunteer Program in a State Mental Hospital," in *The Patient and the Mental Hospital*, ed. M. Greenblatt, D. J. Levinson, and R. H. Williams (Glencoe: Free Press, 1957), pp. 593–603.

3. V. A. Gelineau, "Explorations of the Volunteer Role: The Case Aide Program at Boston State Hospital," in *Mental Health Volunteers*, pp. 35–44.

PART III

Education and Research

CHAPTER 8

Psychiatric Education

By Myron R. Sharaf

Of the various educational efforts at Boston State, the training of psychiatrists was at the forefront of concern during the four years this book covers. Although we will, in the following, focus on the instructional program for this discipline, it will be seen that the content and quality of curricula for other disciplines were closely linked with the development of the psychiatric resident's education.

The significance of psychiatric education at Boston State had strong historical roots. One of the key aspects of Dr. Barton's reorganization of the hospital was the establishment of a strong training program for residents. By the late 1940s, the hospital was far ahead of most mental institutions, public or private, in offering the kind of program that would attract the ablest young physicians entering the field of psychiatry. Consonant with the Freudian psychological revolution, which was picking up momentum at that time, the curriculum stressed the study of psychodynamics in general and individual and group psychotherapy in particular.

This brief statement hardly conveys the depth of the impact of dynamic psychiatry on an institution such as Boston State, with its large number of "untreatable" patients. The new teachings brought a feeling of hope that patients could be understood and treated with a rational design. There was hope, too, that some kind of order could be imposed on the overwhelming task of dealing with several thousands of long-term inpatients and many hundreds of new admissions each year.

The preceding should not be taken to mean that during this period the residents did nothing but practice psychotherapy. On the contrary, their service demands were both heavy and exacting. A typical program for a first-year resident consisted of a four-month stint of managing a ward of about thirty acute male patients; four months on a geriatric or long-term chronic service, with many more than thirty patients to manage but usually few new admissions to work up; and four months on an acute female ward. On each assignment, the resident worked under the direction of a senior psychiatrist.

Although the resident assumed an apprentice role in learning from his senior such skills as diagnosis, formulation of treatment plans, and management of patients on the ward, the cardinal teaching emphasis was on individual therapy with a selected few patients and on supervised group therapy. As a result, the resident could not give as much attention to the patients on his ward as he might have wished. Caught in the bind between learning and service, he was encouraged by senior staff to give first priority to education as they conceived it.

It should be noted that the overall values of the training program meshed well with the resident's own career aspirations. Most young psychiatrists at this time in good resident-training programs were principally interested in learning how to practice psychotherapy in the private office or in outpatient settings. If they were interested in teaching, it was primarily supervision of younger psychiatrists learning the same kind of psychotherapeutic skills they valued. Acute psychotic patients at a state hospital were considered far more amenable to psychotherapy than chronic ones and, as teaching cases, far more rewarding. Indeed, some psychiatrists believed that they provided a better introduction to psychodynamics than neurotic outpatients since they illustrated unconscious mechanisms far more dramatically and immediately.

We emphasize this psychotherapeutic ethos because of its importance in understanding many of the later controversies about the resident-training program. In 1963, a solid, committed cadre of skilled teachers, trained during the 1940s and 1950s, shared this ethos and were strongly opposed to anything they regarded as undermining it. The subsequent development of an expanded philosophy of training was to create a painful, if fruitful, period of change in the whole concept of the education of psychiatrists as well as other mental health professionals at the hospital.

We should mention one further point concerning the ideology of the pre-1963 period. There had been a strong emphasis on what may be termed bureaucratic, impersonal standards, or "fairness," especially in regard to the distribution of "scut work," such as service on the chronic and geriatric wards and night and weekend duty. In an economy of scarcity—large number of patients and relatively few residents—life was considered more bearable if the burdens were equally shared or if preferential treatment was granted in terms of clear-cut extrinsic criteria, such as second-year residents having fewer unpleasant tasks than newcomers. Indeed, so deeply engrained was this point of view that many senior psychiatrists preferred an unfilled resident post to having it occupied by a person not performing to the letter the traditional requirements of the position.

To summarize the essential aspects of resident training during the 1940s and 1950s: psychiatric staff and residents by and large shared a common psychotherapeutic ideology and respected their clinical leader. The prodigious demands of a large state hospital were somewhat mitigated by establishing an oasis for treatment within the hospital (the reception building) and then further breaking it down by selecting just those patients for psychotherapy who seemed most amenable to this approach. Service demands or pressures were also mitigated by the aforementioned standard of sharing the burden equally.

Although this situation was in many ways conducive to high morale, the limitations were also great. Chronic patients tended to be neglected and other than the dynamic aspects of psychiatry were scanted in the teaching and training programs. Ward management and psychopharmacology were taught only on the wards by senior staff in charge of a service and then in a somewhat hit or miss fashion.

Even the strong points of the training program began to suffer after 1958, when a highly admired clinical director left to join another institution. Around the same time, competition for residents was developing with increasing tempo from the smaller university training centers, which were starting new programs and enlarging their resident staff. In the country at large, the number of approved residencies was outnumbering the number of applicants by four to three, and many first-class programs were having trouble filling vacancies.

Strictly as a center for training in psychotherapy, Boston State had a very difficult time in the face of this competition. At a smaller center—for example, a general hospital with a fourteen-bed psychiatric unit—residents could carefully work up *all* their new admissions and follow most of them in psychotherapy. Since there were ample residents, all suitable patients, not just a fortunate few, could be treated by this modality. And if the patient were not suitable for intensive treatment, he could at least be seen several times a week in the early stages without the resident feeling that he was neglecting many others if he did so. The resident in a smaller center also did not have to face the formidable obstacles of bureaucratic red tape and overcrowded working conditions.

Thus, it was one thing for Boston State in the 1940s and 1950s to get the jump on its competitors by emphasizing psychotherapy at a time when few mental hospitals, large or small, had the courage or foresight to do the same. It was quite another thing to continue almost exclusively in this direction when other training centers were doing the same but could provide extra advantages —a small case load, a university community, and an unhurried atmosphere. How then was the state hospital going to attract good psychiatric residents under these competitive conditions?

A possible answer to this question was contained in the shifting mood of psychiatry during the early 1960s. Hollingshead and Redlich[1] had demonstrated the neglect of hospitalized lower-class psychiatric patients. Other investigators had pointed to the greater incidence of emotional disturbance among the poor than among the middle class.[2] A host of studies was illuminating the significance of the total hospital atmosphere in affecting the care of the mentally ill. Some investigations were highlighting the need for preventive psychiatry and for more transitional facilities for treating people in the community. Gradually, a new psychiatric zeitgeist was developing, not against the old, but pointing out fresh directions. In the country as a whole, attention was turning to the poor, the black, the "other America."[3] The federal government was prepared to finance all kinds of facilities for the poor, but not programs directed to the already relatively well-cared-for middle class.

Boston State was in a position to convert some of its seeming disadvantages—its large number of poor people and its complex social organization—into training opportunities that would fire the imagination of the young psychiatrist, just as psychodynamic training had excited his counterpart in the previous decade. Dr. Barton had recognized this and had taken steps, such as the home treatment service, to explore new directions. However, the training program as a whole was still far more concerned with maintaining its past traditions than with reaching out toward new horizons that might have made Boston State stand out from other excellent but traditional training institutions.

The Period of Transition: Early Challenges

Of immediate urgency, then, in early 1963 was the state of the resident-training program. The new administrator saw the slackening of interest in Boston State as a preferred place for psychiatric education as a serious threat to the institution. Soon after his arrival he quickly raised a distress signal to both staff and the board of trustees, apprising them of the gravity of the situation.

Another step that spring consisted of a personal effort by the administrator to see if there were still residents searching for a place of training who would utilize unfilled positions for the year beginning July 1. This act reflected a sense of urgency and served as an antidote to the wait-for-next-year philosophy that often affects flagging training programs, as well as declining political organizations.

To find candidates at so late a date, he went first to the most available source—general practitioners who had already applied to Boston State, but had been turned away. Some of these candidates were physicians who had been in practice for some time and now wanted to enter the specialty of psychiatry. Fortunately, their interest was facilitated by a special National Institute of Mental Health grant which provided a substantial training stipend. Some senior staff felt strongly that these applicants were "too old to learn" and particularly too mired in the active, doing role of a general practitioner to adjust to the nondirective explorative mode of functioning of the psychiatrist. Further, they distrusted the motivations of many of these applicants and suggested, for example, that they were bored with general practice and were interested in psychiatry only as an escape rather than as an intellectual endeavor. Such objections notwithstanding, several general practitioners were accepted as residents that July.

It had been customary for a candidate to be interviewed by several senior psychiatrists who would inform him of what Boston State had to offer and would consider his suitability for the program. Some interviewers behaved in a way no longer appropriate to the current situation. They presented the program on a take-it-or-leave-it basis, as though the hospital were still a highly sought-after educational center. At the same time, they themselves communicated little enthusiasm for the program since an underlying depressive note reflected their awareness of the reality that Boston State was not the place it once was.

In his interviews, the superintendent injected a more welcoming note. For example, if the candidate was at the third-year level, he indicated his readiness to tailor a program to fit his particular needs and interests. Here again, as with the selection of residents, there was considerable opposition from most staff members, who wanted all candidates in the first three years of training to follow a more or less prescribed program.

A major effort was then directed toward enlarging the number of applicants. The superintendent very early appointed a committee of psychiatrists to prepare a brochure describing the basic training program. Although this booklet concentrated on the traditional aspects of the curriculum, prominence was given to newer and broader learning opportunities, such as the day hospital, outpatient clinic, and to the possibility that each resident in his advanced training could pursue the path most suitable to his career plans.

The superintendent directed his office to compile mailing lists of potential candidates, even including medical school seniors, who not infrequently began to consider where they would take their residencies even before they started their internships. He made use of his own large network of professional contacts to inform persons in touch with potential residents or residents wishing to transfer of the advantages of Boston State. He also asked friends at top-level training hospitals to refer their overflow candidates so that Boston State could consider their suitability to rebuild its own program.

The reader may ask why *was* the recruitment of psychiatric residents treated with such urgency and given such high priority? Could not senior staff working largely with nonmedical personnel supply good patient care?

Some mental hospitals do in fact provide excellent patient care without any resident-training program. Staff are then spared the many dislocations, the investment in time, and the constant wear-and-tear of having to educate new psychiatrists who usually go on to other pastures just when they have acquired skills that make them valuable to the hospital.

At Boston State, however, there would have been grave disadvantages in not having a good educational program. First, young psychiatrists, like other students, bring fresh ideas and critical minds to a large state institution, thus enlivening an atmosphere which can easily become stultifying and routinized. Second, residents who have had a rewarding learning experience are prospective candidates for permanent staff positions. Finally, for an institution like Boston State, located in an urban area with many excellent competing mental health facilities, lack of a program, or a poor program, militates against the recruitment of good personnel at any level. Since the psychiatrist occupies the top of the hierarchical pyramid within the mental health professions, members of other disciplines, in evaluating hospitals and clinics, place great weight on the quality of psychiatric staff. Pertinent also to Boston State was the fact that its senior staff were particularly interested in teaching, and in teaching able young psychiatrists. It would have been utterly demoralizing to senior staff to abandon the program altogether or to give it a low rating among hospital priorities.

A final practical point was that, in 1963, leadership posts in mental health were almost entirely occupied by psychiatrists. At that time, if Boston State wanted to conceive of itself as training future leaders, it had to concentrate on psychiatric residents. Since then, in Massachusetts as elsewhere, qualifications for leadership have broadened. Now psychologists, sociologists, social workers, and nurses can hold high-level positions. In fact, nonmedical personnel with appropriate training and experience may become superintendents of state hospitals or schools for the retarded. Only a relatively short time ago this policy would have been boldness in the extreme.

We emphasize these considerations not to get into any debate about the role of psychiatrists vis-à-vis other mental health professionals. Rather, we wish to underscore the complexities surrounding the nature and timing of change in a large organization highly sensitive to vibrations in the professional atmosphere. Even if the superintendent, in 1963, had had a strong desire—which was not the case—to play down resident training and advance other kinds of education, it still would have been unlikely that he could have succeeded given the conditions that prevailed in psychiatry generally at that time and at Boston State in particular. Innovations require some discontinuity with the past; otherwise they are not innovations. But they also require some continuity, lest they be so disruptive that they wind up as bizarre experiments, devoid of any widespread support inside or outside the institution.

The same issue of continuity pertains to the superintendent's administrative decision to concern himself first of all with recruitment. Traditionally, the superintendent at Boston State had been more directly involved in this aspect of the program than, for example, in curriculum development, direct teaching, or clinical supervision of residents. As we have indicated, the new administrator did have his disagreements with staff about who should be selected for training or what kind of special programs would be arranged for particular residents. However, in general, the recruitment area was a "soft" one in terms of institutional change, a question of filling a vacuum rather than of reallocating existing lines of authority. Administratively, there is wisdom in a new leader devoting himself first to such neglected but important "soft" areas rather than to entering immediately the thickets of controversial areas where staff's feelings are highly charged.

It is interesting to note that few psychiatric staff care to take on the onerous task of organizing large mailings to prospective applicants. Few care to write letters to friends informing them of the merits of the program at the hospital. Most professionals consider this kind of chore as grubby and dismal and perhaps a bit denigrating. By energetically fulfilling this commission, however, the superintendent visibly underlined his right to exercise one of his prerogatives: to play an important, decisive role in the selection of residents. His assumption was that how he used this power could radically affect the whole future direction of the hospital.

Some discussion is also necessary in regard to dissensions created by administration's policy of tailoring programs to match particular residents' needs. We have mentioned the value assigned by certain of the teaching staff to equal treatment for all. In addition, senior staff placed a premium not only on individual and group psychotherapy but on residents going through prescribed rites of passage considered to be fundamental to all psychiatric clinical understanding—experience with acute cases, chronic cases, geriatric patients—all within the psychonanalytic conceptual framework.

Inextricably mixed with this philosophy were mundane practical considerations, for many of the senior psychiatrists who taught the residents psychotherapy were also in charge of active services. They wanted residents to help with the many clinical tasks inundating their personnel. Residents' help was particularly critical on admission wards, which handled about twenty-five hundred admissions per year. From the point of view of those on the inpatient firing line, resident manpower was viewed as much more important than manpower for less heavily burdened new community services.

However, from the applicant's viewpoint, the community services were often among the more compelling reasons for coming to the hospital, especially for residents beyond the second year of training. From administration's viewpoint, it was better to have a resident on a day hospital service than to have no resident at all, yet it was often difficult to convince some staff of the validity of this simple point. By making exceptions and individualizing the program, residents could be recruited who could not have been recruited under other conditions, and, given a sizeable number of residents, funds for education and other purposes could more readily be obtained, which in turn would increase the attractiveness of the institution to other potential trainees. When this plateau was reached, it would then be possible to become more selective in the appointment of new residents, even returning to a less individualized system of resident placement if one so chose.

The same kind of thinking applied to the selection of special residents, such as the general practitioners about whose capabilities there were many doubts. If one waits for excellence in order to begin, one may never get the show on the road and incidentally perhaps never attain excellence. Moreover, the superintendent had his own questions about the meaning of "excellence" in psychiatry, as then defined, and wanted at least on a trial basis to see what a variety of different individuals with diverse backgrounds could bring to the hospital and eventually to the field.

Delegation of Authority

We have so far emphasized the role of the administrator himself in providing momentum toward the expansion of the resident-training program. It should be pointed out, however, that from the very start he made deliberate efforts to include many individuals in the planning. As one move in this direction he appointed a psychiatric executive committee, which was largely concerned with issues of resident training. This committee met regularly every week and included, besides himself, the senior clinical director, the assistant superintendent, and two junior clinical directors.

The initial collaboration between the superintendent and the teaching staff was fraught with problems. In developing new programs, such as the rehabilitation service, the superintendent was working in a generally fallow area, with a cadre of new people who shared his philosophy and goals. In the resident-training program, however, creative steps had to be taken in some kind of concert with a group of strong senior staff quite committed to their own way of doing things and resistant, if not antagonistic, toward any major changes in an educational system they themselves had played a large part in designing. Moreover, they had the ideological and personal support of many junior staff whose mentors they had been. Thus, in this program, the superintendent confronted problems similar to those in the crisis of unitization, and both changes reverberated through the entire hospital organization.

One might suggest that the new administrator could replace his teaching staff with men of his own choosing and his own ideological persuasion. Indeed, he could if (1) such persons were readily available, (2) the consequences on hospital morale generally were not too destructive, and (3) he was not particularly concerned about the careers and personal investment in the hospital of the men he would replace. None of these "ifs" applied in this situation.

One might also suggest that short of such replacements, the administrator had to choose between either supporting the present staff in their own directions or ordering them to perform differently. The first alternative was not feasible since the training program could not simply be left alone if for no other reason than it was failing, and failing badly. The second alternative also faced severe problems: orders could have been issued, but as Chester

Barnard has pointed out,[4] the real authority in relation to an order rests with the one who receives it, since it is he who decides whether he will carry it out in a way that fulfills its spirit as well as its letter.

Given these dilemmas, the superintendent pursued a middle course of trying to influence psychiatric staff to accept his views. He also delegated responsibility to them, without at the same time being completely prevented by their opposition from taking various steps of his own. Nonetheless, the senior clinical director, who was in charge of the training program, protested the superintendent's "meddling" in the director's department and openly opposed the movement of the hospital generally toward social and community psychiatry.

The superintendent continued to play a very active role in revitalizing the program although criticism of his interfering continued to be heard. However, we believe that the middle path of trying to preserve what one could from the past and at the same time forging ahead on new fronts made good sense. It allowed room for central initiative, without riding roughshod on the feelings and wishes of senior staff. Very often a new administrator's broom sweeps clean, sometimes too clean; not only the moldering dust vanishes, but a large portion of solid structure as well. On the other hand, too much respect for the existing structure can lead to organizational immobility, with the new enthusiastic leader paralyzed by the resistance around him.

The new leader's enthusiasm is itself an important organizational force. Many studies of institutions focus on the importance of the administrator's taking into account all the various organizational conditions confronting him before moving ahead. They emphasize the difficulties of change and the frequently destructive consequences of too rapid a change. But they often do insufficient justice to the psychology of the leader himself. He must take certain actions early in his tenure. Only when he is fresh to the job will certain needed steps be vividly clear to him. And only in the early period, charged by the challenge of his new responsibilities, will he have the energy and will to accomplish these changes. After a while, he too becomes "acculturated." Like the rest of long-term staff, he may sigh over the sad inevitability of conditions which, in his earlier days, he would have been determined to change. The sheer wear and tear of difficult leadership tasks also makes him less willing over time to take major steps in the face of obstacles.

Building Up Cadres of Support

The ways the superintendent dealt with the opposition depended on the kinds of support he could muster from within the institution and from the psychiatric community at large. In this connection, the administrative diagnosis of the strengths and weaknesses of particular staff members was especially important. Some of the younger staff members were actively involved in community-oriented programs, such as the day hospital and home treatment service, which were not only forging new directions in patient care, but offered excellent training opportunities as well. Over considerable opposition he insisted that, starting in July 1963, third-year residents, and whenever possible, second-year residents, be assigned to regular rotation on these services as well as to more traditional outpatient work in long-term intensive psychotherapy.

The assignment of residents to the newer, more community-oriented services served a dual purpose:

One, it helped break the rigid rule that the basic training experience be confined to inpatient work and psychotherapy with carefully selected outpatients. This very practical measure was in keeping with the broader winds of change which were sweeping over psychiatry in the early 1960s. In this new view, residents should be exposed fairly early in their training to a wide range of therapeutic modalities useful in handling patients in diverse settings.

Two, it helped strengthen the services themselves since the presence of residents brought these new programs additional life and interest. Also, symbolically, the assignment of residents signified that the superintendent had put a further stamp of approval on these innovations. This combination increased the already strong interest of nonmedical personnel in community-oriented functions.

Gradually, the superintendent recruited new psychiatric staff who shared his concern with increasing the breadth of resident training and improving its content. The resignation of the assistant superintendent during the first year of the new administration allowed the appointment of a successor whose overall orientation has been described in the chapter on work therapy. Sometimes formally, more often informally, the assistant superintendent became involved in encouraging and supervising residents interested in programs relating to social psychiatry. The education of residents interested in the treatment of the young was greatly enhanced by the establishment of the adolescent unit during the second year of the new administration.

We might also mention that in that same year a senior psychiatrist proficient in family therapy also joined the staff and suggested that his specialty be a regular part of the resident's required instruction. This proposal was unacceptable to the clinical director in charge of in-service training and for this and other reasons, the family therapist did not remain long at the hospital. However, ideas he originally championed, such as the significance of family therapy and the suitability of diverse kinds of professionals to practice it, were to prevail at a later date. This incident illustrates that men who feel they have failed in instituting a new idea or technique may have paved the way by their very failure for someone else to succeed at a more opportune time. The later practitioner is accepted in part because his predecessor had acted as a lightning rod and permitted some of the angry feelings about a new program to be discharged and worked through.

In piggyback fashion, energetic and successful preliminary steps toward recruitment and program development helped the hospital obtain two federal training grants by July of 1964. One brought funds for increased supervision and education for residents in the basic three-year program; the other provided stipends and supervisory funds for resident training in social and community psychiatry for fourth- and fifth-year residents. In effect, the reorganized basic curriculum and the totally new (for the hospital) advanced training program in community psychiatry had received the federal stamp of approval.

These grants also permitted the superintendent to hire a social scientist who had the dual role of studying the educational processes in resident training and participating in program development in the area of social and community psychiatry. In the course of his research, he interviewed all the residents and many of the senior staff, participated in staff conferences and committee meetings, and reported his findings to the psychiatric executive committee. His observations and analyses became a significant instrument in planning further changes in the training program.

Enlarging the Program

In terms of enlarging and improving the content of the resident-training program, there were at least two important aspects that had to be developed further. The first need was for more centralized didactic seminars in which residents' groups could be brought together for formal instruction. The second need was for daily, ongoing supervision at the ward level.

The first was easier to implement than the second. One can more readily bring in persons with specialized knowledge and experience to give a series of seminars to a group of residents than find supervisors capable of educating residents in ward management throughout the many units on which they served. The reader will recall, for example, that it took considerable time before the adolescent service could amass sufficient staff so that it could assign a consultant to each unit.

In addition to the manpower problem, there was the sociopsychological problem of introducing new teachers within the units themselves. Although every service cried for additional manpower, each wanted the new personnel to fit into existing ways of doing things rather than to communicate new concepts and modes of functioning.

One of administration's important goals was to develop a

stronger educational program in milieu therapy and social psychiatry, a goal much more easily articulated than achieved. We have mentioned the relative ease of introducing new courses as compared with expanding teaching at the unit level. However, their introduction posed its own administrative issues. When we wanted to include a seminar on social psychiatry as part of the program for first-year residents, the suggestion was strongly opposed by the clinical director in charge of in-hospital resident education. He gave several reasons for his opposition: the residents were anxious at the beginning of their training and should not be exposed to too many new ideas at once; they should first get a thorough grounding in individual and group dynamics; a course in social psychiatry would be better scheduled in the third year of training, after the resident had acquired his bread-and-butter skills in psychiatry.

At issue here was a basic disagreement as to what in fact represented the bread-and-butter skills to be covered in the core curriculum. This controversy was not confined to Boston State, but was at that time beginning to flare up in psychiatric training centers across the country. One viewpoint, represented by the clinical director, envisioned the core as intensive exploration of the individual patient which could then slowly radiate outward to groups, families, communities, and so on. The other viewpoint stressed the need for an eclectic curriculum right from the beginning of the resident's education. According to this latter idea, if residents were trained at the outset primarily in psychodynamics, the early imprinting, far from preparing them for work in other areas, such as hospital administration or community psychiatry, might actually hamper their ability to absorb new thoughts and perspectives.

The superintendent chose not to make an Armageddon out of the controversy over the proposed course in social psychiatry for first-year residents, although he was urged by some to do so. Once again, total hospital morale and regard for the highly valued clinical director were important considerations in avoiding a head-on clash. Instead, both the superintendent and the medical executive committee accepted the clinical director's compromise plan to give the course first for *senior* psychiatrists, and later for residents. The ostensible reason for this suggestion was that these men had had little organized exposure to concepts of social psychiatry themselves and should first become familiar with the material findings of that orientation. The compromise plan also "protected" residents from early systematic exposure to these "new" ideas before the senior staff understood in detail what was going to be fed to them.

The seminar for senior staff began in the fall of 1964. It met every other week alternating, symbolically, with another seminar for the same group on the psychotherapy of the psychosis. The course began with a focus on classic studies from the literature which, aside from their own intrinsic value, also provided a relatively comfortable way of getting into a discussion of controversial issues then raging within the hospital. These included the administrator's emphasis on the reduction of the hospital census; the relative merits of nursing homes versus the state hospital for geriatric patients; the suitability of analytically oriented psychotherapy for lower-class patients; the feasibility of psychiatric efforts toward primary prevention, and so on. Thus, the seminar discussion actually took place on two levels: the ideas or programs described in the literature were dealt with academically, but at the same time, open or veiled judgments were expressed as to their wisdom or feasibility at Boston State. The fact that the superintendent often attended the seminar meant that it could be used, at least obliquely, by some seniors as an opportunity to let him know their opposition to one or another of his programs. This was done through a presumably impersonal and intellectualized examination of similar programs undertaken at other institutions. On the other hand, the seminar permitted the superintendent and his supporters to buttress their viewpoints and program plans with illustrations from the literature.

The seminar leader made a serious effort to integrate social-psychiatric and psychodynamic concepts and approaches. Initially, this was not entirely successful. In an institutional sense, the social-psychiatric position was the insurgent one, no matter how integrated the style of its presentation. Although everyone could agree about general principles, such as providing "good" patient care through "flexible" treatment approaches, in concrete policy issues there were real differences of opinion. Arguments centered about such questions as short- versus long-term hospitalization, breadth versus depth in the deployment of treatment resources, the importance of volunteers, and the value of consultation to community groups. Sometimes it seemed that the seminar simply provided an opportunity for staff members with divergent views to trot out their standard arguments without really listening to those who disagreed with them.

Only in retrospect do many of the values of such discussions appear more clearly. The seminar did familiarize its participants with concepts which originally may have seemed foolish or outrageous. One way these ideas became more acceptable was through their conjunction with others that sounded even more outlandish. Thus, one senior who had originally been quite unresponsive to ideas about milieu therapy became far more interested when he read and discussed concepts pertaining to primary prevention. In contrast to some of the notions in the latter area, milieu therapy suddenly seemed rather benign.

The senior seminar stimulated interest among other staff members in formal instruction in social psychiatry. The first pressure in this direction came from nonmedical personnel who rightly pointed out that many others besides psychiatrists were involved in milieu therapy and social programs. In response to this request, we started a biweekly discussion group for all interested personnel, medical and nonmedical.

Organizationally, this course represented an important innovation since it was the first interdisciplinary seminar at the hospital. Hitherto, and in the main for some time after, courses were organized rather strictly along professional lines. Residents met with residents, psychologists with psychologists, and so on. Even the relatively few in-service training programs for nurses and attendants maintained this strict departmental format. Each professional group was eager to attend a seminar given for a higher-status department, but since each also felt "contaminated" if lower-level staff appeared, it was often difficult to cut through professional barriers.

The interdisciplinary seminar was offered as an elective course. This plan made it more acceptable to the clinical director and other senior psychiatrists since it was not a forced encroachment on the resident's time. Repeatedly, this issue of "protecting" the resident's time would arise whenever a new course was suggested. Not only were the clinical directors concerned about "diluting" the resident's education by too many course requirements, but they were also worried that the residents would neglect their service responsibilities if the academic curriculum was unduly broadened or diversified.

Very gradually, the social-psychiatric seminar became a part of the resident curriculum. At the invitation of the clinical director, a biweekly seminar was started in 1965 for second-year residents, the first such inroad into the basic residency program. Around the same time a course (to be described later) was started in community psychiatry for fourth- and fifth-year residents.

However, it was not until July 1967, shortly after the superintendent left, that attendance at a formal course on the concepts of social and community psychiatry became a requirement for all first year residents. In other words, it took almost four years, despite administration's quiet but unremitting pressure, before education in social and community psychiatry was fully accepted as an integral, essential element in the basic residency program.

One might argue that a more forceful administrative policy could have accomplished the changes in a shorter time. Indeed, it might have, but given the resistances there is no way of knowing at what cost. What we can say is that the changes at Boston State, slow as they may have been, were accompanied by quite tumultuous disagreements and often involved shifts in power that created hard feelings. Still, the developments took place without the resignation of a single valued teacher in psychodynamics inherited from earlier days. Also, there were very few "internal migrations," that is, when a valued individual remains nominally in his former position but is in fact alienated from the mainstream of hospital activities.

The Psychiatric Resident

Before considering further developments in training let us describe what the psychiatric residents themselves were like, what their career aspirations were, and what they expected from Boston State.

A major educational and administrative challenge to the resident-training program was posed by the residents' diverse interests, scholastic backgrounds, social classes, ages, and stages of training at entry. Some were coming to the hospital for their total basic residency; others for a twelve-month stay, not out of choice but because a year at a state hospital, with its great variety of patients, was prescribed by the neighboring university training centers to which they were attached. Residents who selected Boston State as a training site also included older general practitioners and students from foreign countries, who were attracted to Boston State because of its reputation in their native lands. Among the young, American-born residents, the range was wide. Some came with excellent backgrounds and chose the hospital because its educational opportunities matched their interests; others came because they had been turned down at the hospitals of their choice.

More than 50 percent of the Boston State residents were Catholic, a surprisingly large figure compared with the very low percentage found among residents in university centers. Distinctive also was the fact that many of the Boston State residents came from working-class families. The social-class factor may help explain why many were relatively vague about their future psychiatric plans. Partly because of economic insecurity, each step on the educational ladder had been problematic. Unlike many residents from Ivy League colleges, who had known from childhood that they were going into some profession, more than a few of our residents had not been sure in high school that they could even afford college.

This then was the amalgam of Boston State residents: some young and bright and particularly interested in new psychiatric directions; others drifting, waiting to see what the hospital could offer them rather than what they could seek from it; older general practitioners, some still eager to learn but others strongly anchored by experience and age to their own ways of doing things; foreign residents with a wide diversity of motivations and career goals; and bright, middle-class, analytically oriented residents on sometimes unwilling rotation from the smaller centers.

This diversity represented not only a problem but also an opportunity. Much has been written about the discrepancy between the middle-class values of most psychiatrists and the lower-class orientations of the majority of hospitalized patients. Here we had the opportunity to work with many residents who themselves came from lower-class families and could therefore be more resonant to the patient's background—his social class, religion, ethnicity, and hard personal struggles.

Foreign residents are often considered a sign of a hospital's failure to attract Americans. In some instances, language and culture barriers are indeed formidable. Yet, at Boston State, it was readily apparent that some foreign residents had much to contribute to a hospital that had a particular interest in social and community approaches and was in the process of developing an eclectic treatment philosophy. The single fact is that many training programs reject foreign residents automatically, no matter how able they may be. Our hospitals would do well to choose such residents over less capable native-born competitors. Moreover, not only can many foreign residents offer the hospital much, but the hospital can take some satisfaction in influencing through its graduates the development of psychiatry in other countries.

As a group, the residents on rotation from the university centers posed the least problems in terms of compatibility with the majority of senior staff, since most of them shared an intense interest in psychodynamics. Indeed, it was often felt that the seniors preferred these bright young affiliate residents to their "own children" and gave them more teaching time. However this may be, because of their relatively brief stay at Boston State—one year—senior staff also tended to write them off in terms of their possible long-term interest in the hospital, believing that basically they were committed to the university that recruited them in the first place. We were to learn, however, that the hospital's competitive position was underestimated in recruiting these residents for advanced training and even for staff positions. Although many of them were initially ambivalent about the hospital, they were to find much that appealed to them. Many were particularly attracted by the opportunity to assume considerable independent responsibility at Boston State in contrast to the highly sheltered, closely supervised mode of learning at the smaller university centers.

Clinical Experiences

The typical first-year resident went through a baptism of fire during the first few months of his service. Green to psychiatry in general and the hospital in particular, he was nevertheless put in charge of thirty or so acute male or female patients in the reception building. Although he received some orientation during the first few weeks as to the various back-up services and departments of the hospital, as well as its rules and regulations, his immediate learning about patients came largely through doing. In other words, the newcomer was figuratively thrown on the ward and expected to be its leader.

This is not to imply that he was completely alone, since he did get some support and supervision from the senior attached to the service in regard to the work-up, management, and disposition of his patients. But the senior had many responsibilities other than ward teaching and was not always available for consultation. Shy, insecure residents were often reluctant to buttonhole their seniors for consultation and so struggled on, relatively alone.

A further problem was that the resident began his training not with relatively well-integrated outpatients but with extremely sick psychotic people for whom the state hospital represented the end of the road. Often they had been previously hospitalized at private institutions or small teaching centers until the center's patience or family funds were exhausted. The resident was often discouraged, to say the least, as he surveyed record after record showing severe longstanding mental illness and many earlier hospitalizations for every aberration ranging from self-castration through acute alcoholism to potential suicide. In contrast to the patients in treatment at smaller hospitals, most of the Boston State population represented the psychological casualties of modern living at the lowest end of the social spectrum.

The complexities of the resident's life were not limited to the patients. As team leader he had to learn to work with ward personnel, particularly the head nurse and three or four attendants assigned to his team. Because of the demands of his ward duties, he was more dependent on them than they on him. In many important ways, the quality of his hospital experience was profoundly affected by whether he was able to enlist his team's cooperation, and they could make his life wretched if he failed to do so.

It should be stressed that the head nurse was often young and almost as inexperienced as the resident since the turnover in this discipline was high. The major continuity on the ward was supplied by the attendants, many of whom had been at the hospital for years and had experienced repeated turnover of residents as well as nurses. Some were jaded, guarded, and cynical about their jobs, no matter how the resident behaved. Others were friendly, cooperative, and thoroughly committed to patient care. A large middle group could bend either way, depending on the resident's skill in bringing out the best in them.

It is difficult to convey the range and magnitude of pressures put on the inexperienced young psychiatrist. Patients rushed to him as soon as he entered the ward, wanting "the doctor" to let them out, contact their relatives, help them sleep, and generally relieve their misery. Although he could not meet many of their needs or even spend much time with them individually, he was still formally and legally responsible for their care and painfully aware of his obligations.

Also, whatever negative feelings ward personnel may have had toward the new resident, he still retained the prestige of "the doctor" in their eyes. Moreover, on many wards, they had to get his permission and written orders to grant the simplest privileges to patients—the right to walk the grounds, to take an aspirin, and the like. To be sure, personnel could set up a situation through various devices to coerce the resident into doing what they wanted done, even decisively influencing such major decisions as transfer of an assaultive patient to a maximum security unit. Much of their real power was wielded informally through complaints, wheedling, highlighting certain aspects of patient behavior, distortion of information, or manipulation of other personnel. It was expected that the innocent young resident would take on the leadership of his ward group while he was still trying to learn the subtleties and complexities of the treatment organization.

It was understandable that residents often wanted to retreat from the maelstrom as much as possible and concentrate on their less stressful off-ward activities. These included seminars and conferences as well as the training program's major emphasis on supervised individual and group psychotherapy. First-year residents were required to see at least two long-term patients a week in psychotherapy, for which they received direct supervision from two different seniors. In their group work, they were required to round up anywhere from six to ten patients, preferably long-term ones, with whom they would meet an hour and a half each week, and to act as recorders for another resident's group. In this, too, they received close supervision from different senior psychiatrists.

The required seminars and psychotherapeutic work were particularly helpful for the passive resident in that they provided definite structure and supervision. Here again the system favored the more aggressive, ambitious resident. Thus, while some residents stuck to a minimum of two patients in therapy, others took as many as five or six and were adept at getting additional supervisors to guide them. They knew how to make good use of the grapevine to find out who the best supervisors were for given types of patients. The adolescent unit, for example, very quickly got the reputation of being eager to provide supervision for residents interested in working with young patients. Some residents took advantage of this from the first day, whereas others left the service not knowing what opportunities they had missed.

Although the residents varied considerably in their commitment to learning about psychotherapy, most found their supervised experiences in this area very rewarding. In contrast to dealing with the pell-mell rush of a ward with thirty or more inherited patients, they could concentrate closely on the few they had personally selected for treatment. Instead of brief corridor consultations with their seniors, often about a ward emergency, they could discuss with their supervisor one patient in depth and over time. They had a chance to catch their breath and to reflect with their tutor about what was going on, not only in the patient but also in themselves.

Important learning experiences often took place in this context. Skillful supervisors were especially helpful in encouraging some of the less sensitive residents to become more aware of their mistakes and of how their own feelings were hampering treatment progress. Thus, one older general practitioner came to realize in the course of supervision that his active medical approach was preventing his patient from discussing his feelings, and that problems in his own life often prevented him from exploring those in his patient's. He subsequently decided to go into personal therapy, a decision fairly common among residents and often precipitated by their contact with good supervisors.

In an interview, one resident, who spoke for many of his colleagues, summarized the educational situation at the hospital in the following way: "In psychotherapy, you learn about the mistakes you've been committing, but in the work-up and ward management of cases or in somatic treatments you have to learn much more on your own."

In a sense, the residents were beginning to demand what the superintendent had wanted for the training system—greater educational push in a variety of directions. In part, the superintendent's emphasis on reducing the census, on slowing down the transfer of acute patients to the chronic wards, on finding alternatives to long-term hospitalization, on motivating patients to want to return to the community, all indirectly put pressure on the resident not to limit himself to the psychotherapies, but to use a variety of treatment methods. In order to utilize them, he had to learn about them and he was beginning to ask for, even demand, such instruction.

Examining the Training Program

Most of the senior staff and residents agreed that there were major problems in the resident-training program. However, the suggested remedies were diverse and often negated each other. Although it had become clear that the residents should not be so involved in routine service tasks and that their program should be truly educational, it was not clear how radical the reorganization should be.

While the superintendent was mulling over different approaches to the problem of distilling a clearer message from the residents themselves, a very capable young resident was sounding out his colleagues about starting their own organization in order to have a formal vehicle for expressing their sentiments and wishes. The superintendent heard of this development and gave it his enthusiastic backing. Thus fortified, the young man took up the difficult task of welding disparate kinds of residents into a functioning group. Within several months, the organization elected its officers and began meeting regularly.

About the same time, gaps in the training program, inadequate performance by certain residents, and rumors that residents were seeking openings elsewhere were being discussed heatedly at the seniors' meetings. In response to the accumulating tension, the superintendent appointed a chairman—a respected senior psychiatrist relatively new to the hospital—to form an ad hoc committee and make a report on the problems of the training program. The chairman selected some old and new senior staff members for the committee along with the newly elected officers of the residents' organization.

Given a broad mandate to survey the residents' educational needs and morale and to come up with recommendations, the committee went about its task with considerable gusto. Interestingly enough, it was the first time that residents and seniors met together in a quasi-official capacity to examine collectively and as colleagues the basic issues of training. All the other groups that had for so long discussed resident education—the psychiatric executive committee, the seniors' group, and a curriculum committee that had functioned sporadically—had consisted only of regular staff members. Looking back, one can see that the development of the resident organization and the ad hoc committee reflected not only a particular crisis at the hospital but also a broader trend of student involvement in educational planning, which was just beginning to develop at universities across the nation. Although the residents were mature men—the average age was thirty-three—there was a tendency for their mentors to believe that they knew what was best for the students. One of the early pleasant surprises was the degree of consensus that could be quickly established between seniors and residents as well as between older and newer staff members, doubtless facilitated by the camaraderie that sprang up in the small, informal meetings held in various members' homes, without the restrictive presence of top administrative staff.

The committee immediately concentrated on the conflict between training and service, which was generally identified as the major problem of the educational program. It recommended that the resident be responsible for approximately one-half of his current case load; that all of his experiences be brought under an educative motif; that stronger supervision from seniors be developed for every part of the program; and that adequate time be allowed for study and reflection. The committee strongly endorsed the unitization plan as one way of reducing the burden of new admissions carried by any one service. It raised the question of who would take over the residents' work when their case load was reduced, and acknowledged that such a change would require a much greater investment by other personnel in tasks now assigned to residents.

A limitation of not more than two new admissions per week per resident would permit tutorial supervision of all case work-ups similar to that given in learning psychotherapy. Whatever the treatment pattern prescribed, adequate supervisory attention would be given to the patient as a total individual and to the integration of the therapeutic efforts of all the staff members in any way responsible for him. The committee also urged that the hospital's growing commitment to diversity in treatment method and philosophy made it imperative to develop a highly integrated leadership pattern for the educational process and to end the war of opposing factions that put teachers and residents alike in the uncomfortable position of having to choose sides.

Less major but still important suggestions included earlier resident experiences in the treatment of neuroses and character disorders, perhaps starting in the first year of training; closer supervision of the resident's role as admitting officer (often an inexperienced first-year resident was required to make difficult decisions without senior counsel); and greater emphasis on the teaching of neurology. Finally, the group suggested that there be a continuing advisory committee of residents and senior staff which would meet regularly and give its recommendations to the superintendent and the director of the resident-training program.

The report was submitted to the superintendent, who suggested that it be circulated among all the residents and seniors. Since the residents had contributed significantly to the report, it generally met with their approval. The reaction was more mixed among the seniors. The clinical directors, while accepting some of the recommendations, were rather suspicious of the report's intent because the committee's chairman was clearly critical of much of the traditional program.

The wide representation of the committee made it impossible to dismiss the report as simply a play for power by one or another ideological faction. As a matter of fact, it expressed so many different viewpoints that no one, including the superintendent, was completely happy with it. Administratively, however, it went very far toward building a consensus about change in an area of boiling controversy.

It strengthened the superintendent's hand on a number of issues he was already committed to and called his attention to others of which he was less aware. It was a good example of the use of ongoing studies of an institution as one method of organizational development, a theme that will be pursued in chapter 9.

The report also demonstrated the interlocking nature of changes in the hospital, with developments in one area having sometimes serendipitous advantages in another. Thus, the committee was able to endorse the idea of unitization in terms of its specific interest—improving the training program—which originally was not one of the major arguments for decentralization. Also, the desire to limit the residents' service load in the name of education reinforced the superintendent's, although not particularly the committee's, goal of raising the status of nonmedical personnel and eliminating strict hierarchical divisions as to who could be a therapist.

It should not be assumed that all the recommendations were readily implemented. On the contrary, several were not really adopted for two or three years. The carefully supervised work-up of all new cases still is an unfilled goal. The important point here is that the report became one tributary in a growing current for change.

It also helped legitimate an important change in the administrative structure of the educational system which the superintendent had long been considering—integrated clinical leadership. The situation could not go on indefinitely as it was then, with the superintendent pressing for change and the clinical directors trying to preserve the status quo. Funds from the federal training program had been available for some time to hire a coordinator for the training program, but the superintendent had not been able to find the right man for the job. The committee's report highlighting the need for a clinical leader in tune with the hospital's philosophy served to quicken the search for such a person, and in July 1966, a coordinator was hired.

Cautiously, to avoid any sudden traumatic shifts in power and also to test out the new person, the superintendent initially kept the job rather vague, although he did emphasize the appointee's role as being that of a coordinator rather than the director of the program. Nonetheless, the appointment signified another major step forward, since the coordinator clearly had an eclectic orientation.[5] For example, during his first year he began an elective seminar in family therapy which later became one of the most popular required courses at the hospital. This course was open to all mental health professionals, another step in a trend toward interdisciplinary education.

The relationship between the coordinator and the clinical directors was quite strained during the first year. The various expansions the coordinator sought—more and varied courses, more interdisciplinary education, more emphasis on total organizational change in order to enhance education generally—were again seen by some senior staff as meddling and signs of power hunger. The clinical directors now argued with the coordinator instead of the superintendent over moot issues. The superintendent still arbitrated certain disagreements, but in the course of a year, the coordinator's ascendancy became increasingly apparent and by June 1967, he was appointed director of resident training.

More relevant to our narrative and to the short-term implementation of some of the committee's recommendations were several further developments during the spring of 1966. One event especially expressed the interaction between central teaching and changes at the unit level. This was the two-day visit of Maxwell Jones, the British psychiatrist whose book, *The Therapeutic Community*,[6] had captured the interest of mental health workers all over the world. Jones's lectures were filled to overflowing, as were the ward meetings he attended to demonstrate more concretely his kind of approach to the therapeutic community.

His visit—to be repeated twice during the next two years—had considerable impact on the hospital. At the time of the first visit, staff were concerned that their once-a-week ward meetings were rather desultory affairs. Jones demonstrated how useful such meetings could be, particularly if they were held daily and with a staff review of what had transpired at the previous meeting. One senior in particular became quite inspired by Jones's approach and set about instituting such regular meetings. Of great significance is that this staff member had customarily allied himself with the more traditional viewpoint at the hospital and furthermore worked in the reception building, which had not been noted for its innovations.

In terms of institutional change, the adoption of an innovation by a member of the old guard often carries far more weight than the pursuit of the same program by a new staff member already viewed as committed to the ideology the change reflects. The former is seen as embracing the new idea on the basis of some kind of objective reasoning and not because of a vested interest. In our example, the particular senior's enthusiasm for ward meetings spread rapidly not only to other sections in his building, but to other units as well.

Another incentive to increased interest in ward processes was the anticipated unitization of the hospital. For some time staff in the reception building had claimed that it was difficult to run ward meetings because the turnover of patients was so rapid. Conversely, seniors on long-term services claimed that their patients were either too sick or too nonverbal for such interchanges to be useful. After unitization, all services would have the mixture of both acute and long term patients so many thought necessary for active and cohesive group discussions.

We might mention one other example of change in ward organization which was stimulated in part by the committee's report. A senior on a long-term service was much concerned with how he could reduce the resident's service load on his unit, particularly after decentralization, when his unit would have to manage new admissions in addition to taking care of a considerable number of chronic patients. Stimulated by previous discussions at seminars and by Jones's visit, he inaugurated a new role for some of his registered nurses and social workers as nonmedical ward administrators for long-term cases. Traditionally, the resident was the administrator even if this meant only a kind of legal fiction in which he wrote the orders for patients, orders which the nurses or attendants often urged him to write.

Even though the residents had complained long and often about their service load, some resented the senior's move to put nurses or social workers in charge of the wards, with the residents serving as consultants about such medical issues as drugs. A few residents refused to take this role, arguing that they would be legally responsible if something went wrong, but would not have the authority to order what they thought right. The senior solved this dilemma by serving as consultant himself to one of the wards run by a nonmedical administrator and getting an interested resident to serve as consultant to another ward.

Again, it was important that this change was instituted by a "traditional" senior, highly respected for his longstanding commitment to psychodynamics. Also, once again, a bold new plan was adopted by other services. As time went on, there was less emphasis on the indispensability of the resident for running a ward and more on what was the proper dosage of service experience to insure his optimum education.

Apparent through the transitional period at Boston State was a kind of two-phased organizational rhythm, which became especially noticeable in connection with the resident-training program. The first phase—one that lasted a considerable period of time—had the following characteristics: Every new proposal met with a series of objections as to why its implementation was undesirable; or persons objected to the new idea not on the grounds that it was undesirable in itself, but that its implementation would require various additional steps that could not be undertaken. This phase might in part be described as the "if only" stage: if only there were more residents, fewer patients, more teaching psychiatrists, and so on.

The second phase involved a many-faceted, functionally interrelated network of changes, with a fairly widespread consensus for the set of innovations. Subjectively, those in favor of the new developments had a sense of things clicking into place, a feeling of real movement at last. Each new idea or program need no longer be fought as a separate battle, but appeared as a logical part of the whole.

The period following the committee's report, the decision about unitization, and the appointment of a coordinator represented the second phase in the development of the resident-training program. Solutions to various problems were beginning to coalesce into a growing movement for widespread change. The diverse goals of a lightened service load for residents, decentralization, and an administrative role for nonmedical personnel began to be seen by many not as separate, discrete items on a "change agenda," each having its own problems, but as interrelated developments, the fulfillment of one facilitating the implementation of the other.

There are multiple aspects of the leader's role during both phases of this sequence. In the initial stage, his promotion of free discussion and debate in various group settings serves several functions: it familiarizes staff members with his views and reasoning about proposed changes; it permits give-and-take discussion of the intrinsic pros and cons of a given change; and it allows for some practical suggestions to emerge in meeting the obstacles to the change—some answers to the "if onlys."

In this way, the administrator gradually creates a climate of opinion that begins to shift the focus from raising objections to providing solutions. One particular proposal may bring in its wake a whole network of solutions necessary to meet the objections obstructing the fulfillment of the suggested innovation. We would stress the importance of the leader's sense of timing—how much time to allow for debate, when to press for closure, when the momentum for interrelated changes can be accelerated.

One way the leader can facilitate the development of a consensus for a set of changes and, with the consensus, momentum for its implementation, is by educating staff about the functional links between their different parts. We have stressed earlier that a leader can rarely get full agreement about a new, important change because of the many crosscutting pressures and interests of different groups. However, a person is often prepared to endorse an idea that lies within his "zone of indifference" if the leader can highlight for him how the implementation of that idea can help bring about another idea that is closer to his heart.

Thus, in the development of the resident-training program,

many residents were not especially interested in such arguments for unitization as the advantage of housing chronic patients with acute ones. However, they were extremely interested in what decentralization might mean for them in terms of a more evenly distributed load of new admissions. Many seniors were apathetic to the plan of enlarging the role of nonmedical personnel, but they acquiesced and prepared themselves to experiment with this extension when they saw its possibilities in terms of freeing the resident for more intensive education.

Training in Psychopharmacology

The development of psychopharmacological education at Boston State represents a cogent example of how many of the previously discussed ideological and organizational issues seemingly unrelated to drug therapy affected resident education in this treatment modality. We have mentioned that in 1963 the majority of the psychiatric teaching staff put as little value on drug therapy as they did on social psychiatry. Although at least half of the patients were receiving psychotropic drugs as a sole form of treatment or combined with other kinds of therapy, psychopharmacology was still regarded as of minor importance, something the resident could pick up quickly and need not be taught formally.

Many of the superintendent's early commitments led directly, and sometimes indirectly, to a greater emphasis on drug therapy. Thus, for example, his stress on reducing the census increased the overall concern for chronic patients, including their receiving appropriate psychotropic drugs. One organizational change reflecting this commitment—unitization—lessened the likelihood of the drug regimen of long-term patients not being reevaluated.

In the two years following the new administrator's arrival, drug therapy increased to include about two-thirds of the patients. Interestingly enough, this increase was accompanied by a *rise* rather than by a decline in verbal therapies, according to a study made by Schulberg and associates.[7] Parenthetically, it is worth noting that the last-mentioned finding violated the common perception of many staff members who believed that the increase in drug treatment would be at the expense of individual and group psychotherapy.

Just as the superintendent's interest in reducing the census was a factor in leading to the increase in drug treatment, so his interest in research played an important role in improving the resident's opportunity to learn about psychopharmacology from knowledgeable senior persons. His prestige as a scientist enabled him to recruit several talented young psychopharmacologists who were interested in Boston State because of its greater-than-usual administrative support in addition to its research possibilities.

These researchers spurred a series of investigations concerning the effect of particular drugs on particular kinds of symptoms. A few residents attached themselves to these projects and thus had the unusual opportunity to learn a good deal not only about the action of specific drugs but also about methodology. However, in a state hospital, research projects, like special clinical services, often tend to become somewhat isolated from service tasks. Regular staff members regard them as privileged sanctuaries, free from the daily wear and tear of clinical life. Indeed, some clinicians often felt antagonistic toward drug researchers because the latters' projects sometimes involved constraints on the management of patients.

The real educational significance of research developments in psychopharmacology came through the presence of persons with a considerable background in drug therapy who, in addition to their research, participated vigorously in the clinical training of residents. One psychopharmacologist organized a biweekly seminar that featured distinguished specialists in one or another form of drug administration.[8] He and other researchers were also available for regular case consultations on clinical problems relating to their specialties.

Training in Community Psychiatry

As we have mentioned, soon after his arrival, the new administrator urged that residents in their second and third year of training have some exposure not only to outpatient psychotherapy but also to the newer community services such as the day hospital, the home treatment unit, and the family care program. It should be stressed that for Boston State staff in 1963, the term *community psychiatry* denoted services to persons designated as patients living outside the hospital. More distinctive aspects of community psychiatry, such as consultation to various community groups— general practitioners, welfare workers, clergymen who dealt with high risk populations—were just in their beginning stages of implementation within the home treatment service. Moreover, as we have noted, it took considerable time for community concepts and approaches to influence the treatment of inpatients within the intrahospital community.

From the learning point of view, one great advantage of the community units over the inpatient services was that they had some control over their admissions. Occasionally the director of a community unit would establish too strict criteria, with consequent underutilization of his service but, in the main, residents were provided with sufficient case experiences for learning without being overwhelmed by practical demands.

The resident also had the opportunity to work in settings of high staff morale. The selection of staff on the community units was often the result of negotiation between the director of the unit and the applicant, rather than simply an assignment by a particular department head. Personnel were often young, eager to work on a job where a particular desire for them had been expressed. Moreover, these new services permitted nonmedical staff to exercise considerable responsibility and independent judgment. The team had to learn how to function with nonpsychiatrists doing most of the direct clinical work and with the psychiatric director serving both as administrative leader and supervisor of his staff.

Indeed, the deep involvement of the nonmedical staff posed some interesting issues for residents assigned to the community units. Consider one example drawn from the community assignment most sought after by residents, the home treatment service:[9]

The resident attached to this unit usually made an initial visit to the patient and his family at their home with a nurse or social worker. The resident participated actively in the diagnosis and treatment plan which was formulated by the total staff with the senior psychiatrist presiding. Often the staff decided that the continued treatment of the patient and his family should be assigned to a nurse or social worker, with the resident perhaps serving as consultant or supervisor, but not seeing the patient again except if a need was clearly indicated.

In such an arrangement the resident did not have the authority he often had on the inpatient wards to make a series of decisions from admission to discharge about the patients assigned to him. On the community services the active involvement of the non-medical staff meant not only that they could be the chief treatment agents, but that in disagreements with a consultant-resident they could turn for support to the senior unit director. The often close personal relations between the director and his permanent staff also made this kind of speaking-up more likely than it would be on the traditional inpatient units where ward personnel showed at least overt deference to residents.

Many residents found the home treatment assignment, including its flexible pattern of role definitions, an exciting learning experience, even though after the initial evaluation they had to follow the patient and his family only at some remove. The team design permitted them to see a multifaceted approach to a case; they learned that a nurse could carry considerably more clinical responsibility than they had imagined and that other caregivers, such as general practitioners or clergymen, could be effectively utilized in the total treatment of the patient.

Other residents found the experience quite disturbing. They felt excluded from the close-knit atmosphere that existed among the regular staff, and they disliked their consultant role when a nonmedical staff member assumed the continued treatment of the case. Indeed, their complaints on this score were similar to the objections of many established psychiatrists to community efforts —namely, that they are insufficiently involved in direct clinical work, their motive for entering psychiatry in the first place.

Some residents were able to learn from this new experience and to alter their style to fit the more egalitarian atmosphere of the special unit. Others were resentful and eager to return to a situation where, according to one resident, "it's clear what the doctor does and what the nurse or social worker does, not where everybody's doing the same thing, the way it is on the home treatment unit."

Generally speaking, it would be a mistake for a community service to adapt its organizational arrangements to meet the demands of certain residents for a more structured mode of functioning. Too much would be lost in terms of the staff's own effectiveness. Moreover, it is an important educational experience for the resident to learn how to function in collaborative team settings. However, the dissatisfactions of some of the residents pointed to the educational need for more careful supervision of their problems in adjusting to a different role on the community services. If a greater spirit of team functioning and decision-making had permeated the inpatient settings, there would have been less discontinuity when the resident was assigned to out-patient units.

Whatever the differences of opinion among the residents regarding the organizational arrangements on the community services, there was quite widespread agreement that their experiences on those units had given them a valuable opportunity to see how very sick persons could be maintained outside the hospital. As one resident put it: "When I was on the inpatient wards, all I saw were the failures of the Home Treatment Service—their patients who had to be hospitalized. I used to scoff at what they were doing. But when I worked there, I could see their successes and some of them were very impressive. Now I'll be much less reluctant about treating very sick patients without hospitalizing them."

In our judgment, these community experiences should be part of the resident's education right from the start of his training. They can help him understand the kinds of concepts and practices that prevent unnecessary hospitalization, a valuable type of learning applicable no matter where the resident is working. Moreover, the resident's early contact with the community could well be extended to include not only sick outpatients and their families but a wide diversity of citizens, particularly those who fall within the high risk categories, and the caregivers working with these persons.

We would add to our emphasis on a multiple-treatment philosophy a stress on the value of multiple, early arenas of training and multiple kinds of persons the young psychiatrist can recognize as proper subjects of his concern or as collaborators in fulfilling his mandate. We would further add that there is great value to a relative simultaneity in the resident's learning these different perspectives, with no single treatment, arena, or patient population being designated as the basic or core experience, leaving the remainder to the inglorious status of "peripheral." We would encourage the breaking down of the rigid distinction of traditional forms of training: first phase = psychotics on inpatient wards; second phase = neurotics in outpatient therapy; third phase = consultation work with community groups, and so forth.

Unitization in principle provided the organizational structure for this multiple approach with a group of staff persons being totally responsible for all phases of therapeutic and preventive work with a specific population. However, it took several years following the partial decentralization we described before there was the beginning of a real synthesis of diverse services within a given unit rather than the more traditional division of separate services for inpatients, outpatients, home treatment cases, and so on. And only with such a cluster of services in a given unit could one think of multiple educational experiences beginning right at the start of the resident's training.

This kind of thinking was fairly abstract compared with the reality of 1963 and the years immediately following. At that time the focus throughout the basic residency was largely on inpatient work, with a few assignments on community services. In order to provide for more extensive and intensive training in community approaches, the superintendent applied for and in 1964 received a federal grant for the training of fourth- and fifth-year residents in social and community psychiatry.

This program was designed to give advanced residents supervised experiences in a wide range of social and community projects. These included: administering a ward along therapeutic community lines; running a day hospital, night hospital, and halfway house; learning to treat such special groups of patients as drug addicts[10] and adolescents; acquiring particular skills in therapeutic modalities such as family and group therapy, which were especially useful in community work; treating patients and their families in the home; and consulting to a wide variety of community caregiving groups.

By specifically designing the program for advanced residents, the superintendent avoided the endless arguments as to what the core training curriculum should be. He also avoided any further embroilments concerning the deprivation inpatient senior psychiatrists felt when basic residents were assigned to the outpatient services. Some controversies remained, however, as to how extensively interested third-year residents could participate in the advanced program. In any case, the existence of such a program could act as a magnet for residents in the basic training program, permitting them to participate insofar as their interests dictated and their other commitments allowed.

The burgeoning federal interest in training psychiatrists for positions of administrative leadership in community mental health centers facilitated the acquisition of the grant for our advanced program. But there remained the acute problem of recruiting residents for a program that had not yet become of primary interest to most young psychiatrists, that offered only a meager federal stipend, and that had as its setting a state hospital rather than a glamorous small university center.

A useful administrative strategy in this situation was to start the program even before the training positions were filled. We encouraged junior staff psychiatrists to consider themselves advanced residents so they could participate in courses and get certain field experiences specifically designed to meet their training needs in administrative and community psychiatry. This format continued to some degree even when the federal training positions were filled. For example, an ongoing seminar in advanced social psychiatry, conducted by the author of this chapter and a senior psychiatrist, included not only those officially enrolled as trainees, but junior psychiatrists and third-year residents as well.

In addition to discussing particular field experiences of the participants, which varied depending on their interests and assignments, this weekly seminar tried to cover common concepts which cut across such different social systems as the family, the hospital, and the community. Thus, the "culture of poverty" could be seen as it affected the state hospital, the community life of an urban ghetto, and the immediate milieu of a child growing up in a disorganized, lower-class family. Such diverse readings as Goffman's *Asylum*, Claude Brown's *Manchild in the Promised Land*, and Minuchin's papers on the family therapy of lower-class patients[11] were used to illustrate concepts drawn from one terrain which were also relevant and applicable to different milieus.

We tried to marshal the same kind of thinking in supervising the clinical field placements of the advanced trainees. Concepts and techniques of community psychiatry could be learned in connection with running a ward as well as through assignment to the home treatment service. It is frequently overlooked that the hospital provides the same kind of challenges that originally inspired the community approach, too many patients for too few psychiatrists, necessitating an increased role for immediate caregivers (in the hospital setting, the nurses and aides); the need often for a greater affinity in social class and general background between "treater" and "treated," be the treater an indigenous community worker, an exaddict, or a hospital attendant; the need to deal with the immediate crisis *in statu nascendi*, be it a crisis in the life of an outpatient or an aggressive outburst on the ward.

At the same time, we were concerned that the advanced resident should have supervised experience in the more distinctive aspects of community psychiatry. By these we mean not only seeing non-hospitalized patients in a variety of settings, but also consulting with caregiving groups who work with high risk populations. We also mean the resident's involvement with enterprises, such as local health centers or settlement houses, that are likely to help provide a stronger sense of cohesion and hope in a disorganized and apathetic neighborhood.

Some advanced residents were prepared to plot the kind of broad pioneering course we had in mind. Thus, one fourth-year resident, with the help of several senior figures, wove together a true social and community program for his entire year's experience. Part of his work consisted in establishing a new day hospital for chronic patients. He developed a thriving service by keeping his admissions open to anyone who appeared to need help. He thus avoided the pitfall of applying the too-strict criteria of many underutilized community services, criteria that few of the emotionally disturbed in our lower-class community could meet: "must have an involved family," "must be in a current crisis," "no history of repeated past hospitalizations," and that old platitude, "good teaching case."

In addition to establishing an innovative service, this resident was also able to make use of ongoing community research projects for his own education. Under the guidance of a distinguished senior researcher, he studied the effect of psychiatric consultation to nursing homes, some of which contained a large number of ex–Boston State patients. He learned not only about the complex methodological issues involved in a rigorous study on the effects of consultation, but also about the equally complex practical procedures and social and political skills involved in gaining and maintaining access to nursing homes which are traditionally suspicious of outsiders they fear may be checking up on their adequacy.[12] He was also a consultant to the family-care program and to a school for the mentally retarded.

While some advanced residents had this varied kind of supervised experience in innovative community enterprises, others preferred simply to get a taste of what were then still considered avant-garde experiences, such as consultation. They would sit in on a seminar for general practitioners or clergymen, or participate for a period of time in the psychiatric department of a neighborhood health center. After this brief exposure, they would return to more traditional kinds of community psychiatric activities, such as individual and group psychotherapy with outpatients, because they felt that their role in the newer enterprises was too vague and unfulfilling.

In short, there was a tendency for some advanced residents to retreat from the innovative aspects of the new programs into older, more established ways of doing things. It was hard for them to make the complex switch from treating patients to community work where the roles of "treater" and "treated" are not so neatly assigned or clearly delineated. Furthermore, many of the most successful practitioners of community skills were still flying by the seat of their pants and had not yet designed a clearly codified, communicable set of concepts and techniques.

Looking back upon our mistakes, one can see more clearly that for a community training experience to be maximally successful, one must either be highly selective in the kinds of residents one chooses for work in a new program, or make every effort possible to push the reluctant young psychiatrist, albeit with careful guidance, into the turbulent waters of community work. For various reasons, some outside our control, we were not always able to meet either criterion.

As time went on, however, the hospital was in a better position to choose advanced residents specifically interested in new areas and to structure carefully supervised experiences for them. We found it particularly helpful to provide each advanced resident his own individual tutor, not only to design a special program for him, but also to help explore the inner and outer obstacles to his greater involvement in community work.

In so doing, we learned that the resident's countertransference is as important in community realms as it is in his therapy with individual patients. Thus, one advanced resident was extremely reluctant to become practically involved in community matters despite his repeated assurances that he desired to do so. Whatever community experiences were offered he would either dismiss as too vague or halfheartedly try and then withdraw. It so happened that this particular resident, an émigré from Eastern Europe, had gone through a long series of childhood and adolescent marginal experiences, including attendance at a sectarian school while most of his friends were in government-run academies. For him, social and community work represented a continuation of his marginal role. He strongly desired to "belong," to be a member of the psychiatric establishment, to practice "regular psychiatry" rather than to explore the somewhat déclassé terrain of community psychiatry.

Certain organizational factors at Boston State, and we believe at other institutions, militated against a psychological exploration of the resident's difficulties in social realms. For one thing, those supervisors most helpful in stimulating the resident's self-exploration often confined themselves to supervising individual or group psychotherapy, since they themselves were not interested in larger social and community efforts. On the other hand, as we have noted, the most enthusiastic proponents of the newer efforts often considered themselves in opposition to the traditionalists, that is, they were interested in community efforts but not in complex intrapsychic factors. Unfortunately, their deemphasis on the intra psychic often interfered with their capacity to help the resident in community areas when the resident's own conflicts were part of the obstacle to his getting involved or to making effective use of himself when he did participate.

Psychiatry's current ideological atmosphere permits or encourages a readier integration of different viewpoints and programs than our administration was able to achieve during our early years at Boston State. The field as a whole is less caught up with bitter polemics about the rank of one or another treatment approach, or about the appropriate arena for the psychiatrist's work, although there still exist major differences of opinion about the importance of primary prevention or the psychiatrist's participation in community organization at the grass-roots level. It may be that we are generalizing too much from the situation at Boston State where a lessening of harsh debates and sharp polarizations did seem to occur. Perhaps the earlier power struggles and ideological divisions paved the way for the later moves toward integration, which would have been impossible without the sometimes tumultuous working through of conflicts.

Reflection

The juxtaposition of factors necessary to get a program started or to lead to rapid, accelerating momentum in a new enterprise after a protracted period of debate, as discussed earlier, requires some further attention.

In the case of the advanced program, there were two important ingredients for the launching of a new enterprise: the right national climate of opinion and a leader who was prepared to initiate the program not only in terms of his immediate interest but also in terms of his longstanding commitments. In addition, there were also some staff persons, either inherited or recruited by the new administrator, who also had a substantial interest in community psychiatry. However, what was lacking was also important. Beneath the superintendent, at the level of top lieutenants, there was only scattered support for active involvement in community matters, a situation that existed throughout the country in the early 1960s and was not unique to Boston State. The leader is often more responsive to the emerging trends than the people immediately beneath him; he *is* a leader in part because his interests match the emerging shifts in emphasis or because he is able to adapt himself to change. However, the field of community psychiatry was still too new for much "bench strength" to have been developed. Those who had risen to positions near the top had done so because of their expertise in traditional modes of psychiatric practice, not because of their pioneering in community efforts.

Another important lack was that the hospital itself was not oriented to community programs. Understandably, its main focus was on its historic mandate—to house and treat the severely disturbed. Even though in the 1950s and 1960s the number of outpatients rose steadily, community psychiatry in its truest sense involved far more than seeing outpatients. As we have noted, it required many, varied, and often tumultuous organizational changes, including but by no means limited to the development of new programs, before even the scaffolding could be created for genuine, widespread community involvement on the part of the hospital.

One final lack in 1963 and the years immediately following was serious "pressure from below" for innovative community psychiatry. By this we mean the demand from students, the incoming groups of residents particularly. We recall that the psychological revolution exploded in resident-training programs in the late 1940s and early 1950s when there was a combination of eager, able teachers interested in transmitting psychodynamic knowledge, and residents, fresh from World War II, demanding such instruction. Starting around 1967 and developing rapidly since then, a demand for community psychiatry training began to sweep the country: medical students and residents in all specialties—but perhaps especially psychiatry—were insisting on a closer involvement of medicine with the community, especially the poor and medically neglected within our midst.

We emphasize the factors favoring and inhibiting the development of programs in community psychiatry at Boston State around 1964 in order to alert psychiatric program directors in whatever area to some of the considerations that must be borne in mind in starting new enterprises. That somewhat hackneyed phrase, "There is nothing more powerful than an idea whose time has come," is relevant here. The life of an innovative leader would be fairly simple if it were always apparent to him and others that the time of an idea *had* come. On the contrary, the leader must take risks with ideas whose time may or may not be around the corner. He may have to endure the uncertainty of facing unanswerable, searching questions about the wisdom of his new programs, questions asked not only by others but by himself as well.

In making his estimates and his list of priorities, he not only draws on his own experiences and psychiatric knowledge as to what is desirable and needed, but also makes careful assessments of his sources of support, present and future. The present ones are more obvious, for example, federal interest in community programs during the early 1960s; the long-range ones require more sensitive and chancy predictions. In retrospect, for example, it seems clear that the social concerns and idealism of college students in the early 1960s would find expression by the late 1960s in the ethos of medical students and residents.

But this was by no means obvious in 1963. Also, more negatively, who could have predicted at that time that the Vietnam war and other sociopolitical developments would lead in six short years to a drastic reduction in federal funds for community psychiatry programs?

In short, once again we would call attention to the need for toughness in the innovating leader, in this connection the toughness to stick to new ideas and programs during the difficult early periods when opposition is more widespread than support. It requires patience and tenacity to persevere with programs that lack wide support from staff and even wide interest from students, to persist without becoming retaliatory in the face of criticism and endless questioning. The organizational pull is always toward the old, the familiar, and the well established. The leader's task is to see beyond the horizon, to be ahead of the institution but not so far ahead as to be out of touch with it. With skill and some luck, he will find himself on a path where other, often initially unsuspected developments are converging.

In the case of education in community psychiatry, it would take the institution several years to "get itself together" to even begin to think of wide treatment and preventive services for catchment areas; it would take time for linkages to be established with other mental health centers, community agencies, and ordinary citizens for such an orientation to appear practical and feasible; it would take time to build up sufficient staff support or to recruit new members; it would take time to develop the appropriate zeitgeist to interest and inspire prospective students. It is the sowing of difficult, not immediately fruitful fields in the early, hard stages of development that is the leader's particular challenge and opportunity.

REFERENCES

1. *Social Class and Mental Illness* (New York: John Wiley and Sons, 1958).

2. J. A. Clausen, "The Sociology of Mental Illness," in *Sociology Today*, ed. R. K. Merton, L. S. Broom, and L. Cottrell (New York: Basic Books, 1959), pp. 485–508; S. M. Miller and E. G. Mishler, "Social Class, Mental Illness, and American Psychiatry: An Expository Review," *Milbank Memorial Fund Quarterly* 37 (1959): 174–99; L. Srole et al., *Mental Health in the Metropolis* (New York: McGraw-Hill, 1961).

3. Michael Harrington, *The Other America* (New York: Macmillan, 1962).

4. *The Functions of the Executive* (Cambridge, Mass.: Harvard University Press, 1938).

5. F. J. Duhl, *A Personal History of Politics and Programs in Psychiatric Training* (forthcoming).

6. (New York: Basic Books, 1963.)

7. "Treatment Services at a Mental Hospital in Transition," *American Journal of Psychiatry* 124 (1967): 506–13.

8. A. DiMascio and R. I. Shader, eds., *A Handbook of Clinical Psychopharmacology* (New York: Science House, 1970).

9. See L. Weiner et al., *Home Treatment: Spearhead of Community Psychiatry* (Pittsburgh: University of Pittsburgh Press, 1967).

10. D. J. Myerson and J. Mayer, "The Drug Addicts," in *The Practice of Community Mental Health*, ed. H. Grunebaum (Boston: Little, Brown, 1970), pp. 197–218.

11. *Families of the Slums* (New York: Basic Books, 1967).

12. B. Stotsky, *The Elderly Patient: Mental Patients in Nursing Homes* (New York: Grune and Stratton, 1968).

CHAPTER 9

Research

By Milton Greenblatt

The mental hospital is at its best when it embodies a therapeutic community, a training center, and a laboratory for the study of human behavior, all developed synergistically and in harmony. Of these three, the last is most often lacking and yet most necessary in order to impart vitality and intellectuality to an institution striving for quality and excellence. Dynamic research organizations are the sine qua non of medical schools and university hospitals, but unfortunately only a few state hospitals have "arrived" in this sense. The vast majority lack the organization, the spirit, the facilities, and the manpower to develop investigations along a broad front.

Boston State in 1963 was better than most. It had in the past carried out research in a number of areas—individual and group psychotherapy, depression, geriatrics, and home treatment, to name a few. However, the projects came and went, usually seriatim, and usually conducted by departments of psychiatry and psychology of local universities. The ideas, programs, designs, methods, money—and the control—were all vested in people or departments outside the hospital. Frequently, Boston State had merely been a place that furnished the clinical material, laboratory space, or just nominal affiliation. Professionals within the hospital cooperated, but were left out of the center of research activity in varying degrees, with little of the joy of a problem solved, of a discovery made. This situation had bred a sense of being exploited, of the hospital being plundered for its resources.

Thus, despite the many investigative studies ongoing over many years, a stable research organization as such had not emerged.

Building a Research Organization

The task of establishing a lively research organization in a large state hospital is an arduous job indeed. Recruitment of personnel with creative interests is exacting and sharply limited. Of those who do make the move, the best find it difficult over the long run to tolerate the intellectual aridity and professional impoverishment of the average state hospital. Unless one is blessed by proximity to an urban educational center, as we were, by affiliations with institutions of higher learning, by training programs for psychiatrists and graduate students of many disciplines, by a tradition of research, by research leadership of experience and broad influence, by generous allotments of funds from state, federal, or private agencies, or, lacking these, by considerable know-how in the area of grantsmanship, the job is well-nigh impossible. Yet, wherever it *has* been possible to develop a significant research organization, the hospital has usually forged ahead in patient care and innovative clinical programs, in professional status, in esteem of the lay community, and in better quality personnel at all levels.

A research organization cannot be merely a building set aside in which a group of investigators pursue studies of interest to themselves or a few others. Nor can it be an activity peripheral to the institution, an accretion upon the hospital system. It must be a vitally coordinated effort to gain new knowledge in which the process, the drama, the thinking, the successes, and the failures are all shared with the larger group.

The spectrum of studies must cover a wide range—some immediately applicable to treating patients, some relevant to the advancement of laboratory knowledge or techniques, and many in between. There must be not only full-time men in the organization—indeed, full-time investigators are the backbone of any research enterprise—but also part-time workers and many others who are doing research in connection with their clinical or administrative responsibilities. And, rather importantly, the therapeutic organization itself, which often escapes serious attention, should be one of the primary foci of the research efforts. Therefore, morale, communication, hierarchy, the changing roles of therapeutic personnel, the evolutional development of new goals and practices for services, and the relation of the hospital system to surrounding systems and organizations come within the scope of important research carried out by the research team.

A research organization does not grow by chance. Someone has to raise funds, carve out space, acquire instruments and apparatus, recruit promising workers, furnish proper conditions for work, including opportunities for continued stimulation, and supervise the relationship of research to education, training, and treatment. It is often vital, too, that a significant person be provided the research workers as an identification object, a model, a status figure: someone to function as "father" to the younger workers, especially when they are in the midst of discouraging turns in their work or distressed over their future careers, or even when they are fighting with each other. Such a person, hard to find, is commonly called a research director—a poor description of the multiplicity of roles he fills. As a matter of fact, what he does *not* do is direct, in the sense of telling the researchers what they should do or asking them to work on *his* ideas. His directing is, in fact, largely the facilitation of their own direction, bringing out the creative potential with which they were born. This person is a benign "father" and painstaking teacher, not an "orchestra conductor" who requires performance consistent with a score that he interprets in his own way. At the same time, he is acutely aware that however much an individual researcher prizes his autonomy and independence, he is also greatly influenced, often unconsciously, by the environment in which he lives and by the people he meets and associates with. It is the director's wisdom about subtle influences affecting the creative person and his ability to alter these conditions in a favorable direction that give him whatever scope he may have in creating the type of research department or organization he dreams about.

The Pool of Potential Talent

Where do the research workers come from who are to build this scientific edifice? Since the research organization will function within the context of a hospital, it would be natural to look first to the medical profession for manpower.

Psychiatrists can contribute almost indispensable values to a research organization concerned with behavior and adaptation of man; so much so that to be without a full-time psychiatric researcher can be a significant handicap. These values are: a broad scientific background, which views the individual as a biological being as well as a psychological entity; intensive clinical experience with a wide array of maladaptations and mental disturbances, plus the clinical judgment that derives from it; and the invaluable credential of a medical degree, which gives him the legal sanction to assume responsibility for a treatment facility, including prescription for the care and treatment of patients. Further, the prestige conferred by the medical degree and psychiatric training often makes his leadership readily acceptable to workers from other disciplines. If, in addition, he has also won his research credentials, he is then, in the eyes of many of his colleagues from related fields, truly fit to lead.

However, only about 10 percent of medical students eventually go into psychiatry, and of these only 3 percent—roughly twenty to thirty per year—choose research per se as a full-time occupation. This is an astonishingly small number to carry the major burden of advancing knowledge in a field so full of speculation, so lacking in new techniques and treatments, so rapidly changing in its orientation, and so overwhelmed with demands for service. To capture a fair portion of these career investigators-to-be is the desire of all medical schools and university hospitals. Think, therefore, how difficult the competition must seem to a large state hospital aspiring to become a research and intellectual center.

If the competition is too great and one cannot recruit full-time psychiatric researchers, it is still possible to build a significant and highly productive research team without them. For far outnumbering the small 3 percent who plan to devote full time to research are the young psychiatrists, often with a research background, who deeply desire a career that combines research with clinical work and teaching. Many of these men have burning questions regarding the etiology of human behavior which they hope to answer within a clinical framework. The clinical and research programs they generate in the course of their endeavors are sorely needed for they may lead the way to many innovations in hospital treatment and practice. Furthermore, in pursuit of combined clinical and research objectives, a well-motivated part-time investigator will often spend many extra hours on his program, so that often two part-time workers may add up to more creative drive and research productivity than one full-time man. Moreover, there are two minds around rather than one, with greater opportunity for interaction, interstimulation, and sociality.

In addition to the above, relatively large expansions of research staff can come from the ranks of psychologists, sociologists, and other behavioral scientists, as well as from basic scientists—biochemists, pharmacologists, geneticists, neuropathologists, neuropsychologists, and many others. The important point is to erect a solid bridge to the university departments in which they are trained so they can move easily to the mental hospital with the expectation that they will find the environment fascinating and the administration cordial and cooperative. As a matter of fact, whereas psychiatrists often contribute something special to research in the field of mental health, the contribution from workers in nonpsychiatric disciplines has been of major significance. It is widely known that for many years the number of federal grants awarded to nonpsychiatrists has exceeded those given to psychiatrists. And probably most of the well-disciplined and methodologically sound studies have come from research teams with nonpsychiatric leadership.

One full-time research psychiatrist and perhaps two or three other psychiatrists giving part time to clinical research projects, as well as a few workers from related disciplines, each pursuing his own direction, can form the nucleus of a solid research organization. Now the group is ready to grow to include others who would like to enhance their role within the hospital structure—nurses, social workers, occupational therapists, attendants. Include also volunteers and physicians from other disciplines looking after the medical and surgical needs of patients and you have a rich pool of talent from which to draw.

The point here is that research cannot be construed as existing only with a capital *R*. Research as an attitude, a questioning spirit, an attempt to gather information, even if in a naïve, unsystematic way, can uncover some very remarkable findings. It will be a long time before the highly specialized, critical-minded, and design-conscious research experts will be able to solve the problems posed by the attendant, nurse, or volunteer. All professionals, indeed all groups involved in care and treatment, should be encouraged to study and analyze their roles and services, with guidance from the research staff. There are numerous examples of highly successful inquiry by social workers, nurses, occupational therapists, rehabilitation counselors, clergy, and volunteers, although, to be sure, few of their efforts reach publication in scientific journals. These people are usually pleased to accept research supervision, and the occasional publication that may come from one of their members raises remarkably the level of esteem of the whole group.

Initial Organizational Steps

Given a foundation of workers in areas of investigation, one can start building a research organization. Our first major effort at Boston State was to find the right kind of people to form a proper nucleus. The administrator studied lists of former students, associates, and collaborators from his twenty-three years at Massachusetts Mental Health Center, during eighteen of which he functioned as director of research, and considered each from two standpoints: his potential contribution as a researcher, and what would entice him to Boston State. In addition, each new person applying for a staff position was scrutinized as to whether he possessed any interest in research or could be developed in this area, even on a part-time basis.

Fortunately, there was no scarcity of talented individuals interested in the research opportunities presented by a large hospital and stimulated by the idea of forming a new research organization. Several former friends and associates were quickly contacted. One young research psychiatrist wanted to develop a sleep and dream laboratory to continue work he had begun at the National Institute of Mental Health. This was made possible by a research career development grant from NIMH; space, equipment, and additional funds were made available by the hospital. His output was truly remarkable. Studies pursued in his laboratory stimulated enormously staff's interest in this new field. His lectures were well attended and with his background he made the most of the relevance of his area to the general field of psychopathology. Eventually, he built up a staff of twelve workers and published numerous papers in addition to an excellent book on the biology of sleep and dreaming.[1]

Another psychiatrist, a resident at a nearby university hospital, chose to spend part of his time doing research at Boston State on geriatric patients, which were in inadequate supply in his own institution. Eventually he became a full-time member of our staff, obtained a large grant for the study of the adaptation of our geriatric patients in nursing homes, built a formidable research team of his own, and published, in addition to a comprehensive book on this subject,[2] many related articles. Both these men were fortunate early recruits because they already possessed considerable research experience and know-how.

A brilliant young sociologist with whom we had worked for many years, a pioneer in the student volunteer movement and in the development of halfway houses, also chose to throw in his lot with us. We concurred enthusiastically with his desire for freedom to push in any direction he wanted and, true to his former style, he quickly gathered around him many inspired students who worked enthusiastically and vigorously in a number of fields. One of the most important developments was the study of families of the mentally ill—based on observations made by his students who began to live with the families of schizophrenics.[3] Soon a psychiatrist interested in family dynamics joined them, and together they established a strong family research center which generated all sorts of ideas, not only for research, but also for training and clinical work. They boldly proceeded to train a variety of people from all professional levels and types in family treatment, and permitted them in turn to train others within their group. A definite shift in the center of gravity from dyad to family was soon noted in the hospital's therapeutic orientation.

As a beginning to the establishment of more basic departments of research, we turned first to the neuropathology laboratory. The routine work of postmortems and tissue diagnosis had so bogged down that laboratory that there was insufficient time to mine the laboratory's rich lode of research material. By contracting out the routine work to specialists around Boston on a consultant basis, we were able to attract a distinguished neuropathologist to head the laboratory. He saw in it the facilities he needed and the freedom to continue the pioneering work he had begun in England, as indicated by the material he most recently published.[4] Since in addition to his expertise in neuropathology, he was also a fully qualified psychiatrist, the advantages to the hospital were doubled. His stimulating discussions on brain anatomy and physiology, his brain cutting seminars, the neuropathologic underpinnings he provided for the newly appointed teachers of neurology, gave this whole domain a bright new glow.

It was obvious early in our program expansion that the whole field of psychopharmacology, including research, needed intensive development. Although we were spending huge sums on psychotropic drugs, there was little training in their proper usage, practically no monitoring of their effects, and precious little research. We were fortunate to be able to persuade a former colleague and collaborator in psychopharmacology at the university center to give a portion of his time to Boston State, where he in turn would find the many chronic patients he needed to continue his work. Moreover, a branch of the NIMH intensive study of the drug treatment of schizophrenia had been established at the hospital and since that project needed additional leadership, he was also asked to involve himself in it.[5] There is no doubt that the work of this man, together with the colleagues he attracted, caused a thorough pervasion of psychopharmacological awareness and interest that had never existed before. The rehabilitation of large segments of the chronic population is owed to their intensification of therapeutic activity on behalf of these neglected patients.

The head of the psychology department, widely known as a valuable contributor to the literature,[6] was nevertheless sharply limited in his research output by the clinical demands of his job. To offset the routine load and to enhance the investigative capacity of his department, he was given a number of stipends in order to recruit other psychologists with research interests. In 1963, his was the only doctorate in psychology at the hospital; by 1967, there were twenty Ph.D.'s working in a variety of fields for whom he could function as the research "father."

The build-up of the psychiatric residency training program, and the general stimulation of training programs in other fields—nursing, social work, occupational therapy, rehabilitation counseling, pastoral counseling, volunteers, and research methodology itself— made it most fitting that the general processes of education should come under scrutiny. Thus a social scientist, long interested in the career development of psychiatric residents, soon joined the ranks to establish still another department. He was another of our congenial and warm collaborators who saw opportunities to broaden his work within a state hospital. He was fascinated, too, by the organizational dynamics of the therapeutic system, and inspired several important studies on management succession, patients' views of the hospital and its treatment program, styles of management, issues in institutional change, and so on.[7]

Along these lines, the Laboratory of Community Psychiatry at Harvard invested heavily in a five-year intensive study of changes in the hospital as it tried to move toward a community center.[8] They assessed periodically the use of various therapeutic modalities by different categories of staff on the patient group, and gave us most valuable feedback on the successful spread of therapeutic efforts to different patient populations as well as on areas of relative neglect. They analyzed unitization and other hospital events, using modern systems theory, and invented new methods of measuring community-mindedness based on methodology used so advantageously by Levinson and others in "authoritarian" and "custodial mental illness" scales.[9]

Space does not permit a full delineation of the many spreading islands of research emphases that came into being during these years, so that at times it seemed that every front of activity was in truth an investigative frontier. Thus the program on the use of volunteers in case aide–type relationships with chronic patients became a fruitful area for investigatory pursuits by social workers; the work program was the research nexus for rehabilitation specialists; the home treatment, adolescent, geriatric, and general practitioner training programs[10]—all became the basis for books that were published under the Boston State imprimatur[11] and the editor who was brought to the hospital to assist personnel striving to piece their observation and thoughts together into some publishable form found herself very busy indeed.

Like any forward-looking business enterprise, the hospital needed "risk capital" to invest in innovative experiments that could help chart the future, even when the chances of reasonable payoff were less than good. Some of this capital came through grants and awards where bold ideas captured the interest of foundations and granting agencies. Even more freedom was possible by the use of state funds in flexible ways. For example, pay blocks for so-called junior physicians were at such a low level of compensation that they were almost impossible to fill. But when offered on a part-time basis to those interested in using their imagination, there were many takers, especially among those engulfed in clinical practice who hungered for the sheer luxury of time to think, read, and invent. This device of part-time opportunities attracted a more adventurous group than the hospital had previously known. And since the opportunities were initially offered on a short-term basis, those who were obviously going down an unproductive avenue soon terminated, whereas those who developed enterprises with promise of future use to the hospital stayed on to pursue their work in an expanded way.

Thus, the new spirit of inquiry, the rewarding of enterprise and experimentation, the expectation of new ideas from every quarter, the use of risk capital, the personal contacts of the administrator and senior staff, the infusion of new personnel, the facilitation of the writing urge not only of research staff but of many others, added to the hospital's training programs, its Boston situation, and its university connections—all these taken together were responsible for a rather formidable research build-up over a relatively short period of time.

The Care and Feeding of Researchers

What are the conditions that will not only attract vigorous, promising researchers to the large mental hospital but, what is more important, keep them there as well?

We might start with the "fecundity of aggregates," the term used by Elmer Southard to express his philosophy of research as a social experience.[12] Gone are the days when the lone researcher pursued his studies in magnificent isolation, appearing only after long intervals to expound his findings to an awestruck audience. In the contemporary scene, we find regular interchange, mutual stimulation, sharing of experience. Seminars in and out of the hospital, meetings with those of similar interests locally and around the world are part of the modern idiom. For the mental hospital, an aggregate of researchers not only satisfies the basic needs of the individual worker for intellectual sociality, but keeps him "in the groove" as well. It also gives strength and identity to the values for which the researcher stands, values complementary to training and treatment.

In the natural course of events, as the research activities grow, several groups of workers aggregate around different themes or disciplines. Yet those interested in neurophysiology can rub elbows and explore common ground with whoever is interested in social organization. The common denominator is the search for ways to understand human behavior more fully and for means to modify disordered lives.

What is the minimum number for that "fecundity of aggre-

gates"? I think it is somewhere between four and eight, depending
of course on the researchers' self-sufficiency as thinkers and workers and on their stage of career development.

It is often difficult for the administrator in a state hospital setting
to assemble even four talented researchers to represent the van-
guard in a previously research-poor organization. Partly, the top
administrator can exert some pulling power if he himself has a
background in research, as already mentioned. But in addition,
other steps are necessary, steps that would not often be required
in a more prestigious academic center. To compensate for the
negative image of the state hospital as a research site, the
administrator must often offer an interested investigator more
than he would in other settings—more freedom, more space, and
more personal support. In addition, to maximize the likelihood of
the initial aggregate being fecund, he would do well to place his
small band of research workers together on one floor of the building. Over time, as the research organization builds up, the necessity for the tight coalescing of the research forces lessens.

In the early days, when the numbers of primary investigators
are few, it is possible for them to come together easily in lunch-
eons, seminars, or evening social-intellectual meetings with a
minimum of effort and a maximum of satisfaction. In these early
days, they have a strong common bond; not only are they few in
number and close to each other, but they differ in several ways
from the rest of the staff, who usually have specific jobs and
routines that do not require too much analysis. The researchers,
however, have the unusual task of reflecting on what they know,
of following ideas to their logical conclusion, of pursuing new
techniques, of adding to the sum of knowledge, and of improving
a body of scientific theory. They also have common problems of
method, money, material, and publication. Thus, to an extent, one
way or another, they are often set apart from the rest of the
hospital.

Later, as the research organization grows and a single seminar
is insufficient to bring the primary elements together with any
satisfactory sense of sharing, new problems develop. It is difficult

for a specialist in social psychology to listen to a long and technical discourse on, say, chemical methodology, without a feeling of frustration or boredom.

There comes a time when the degree of specialization is such that each primary investigator and his department must seek their own colleagues, whether inside or outside the hospital. These trends are necessary and probably good. The only caution is to maintain a high degree of potential for communication between different segments and groups *within* the research department to maximize the possibility of their learning from each other, collaborating with each other, and developing interdisciplinary efforts *intramurally*. If research workers are not encouraged to keep the internal climate in ferment and high productivity, there may be in the long run an attenuation of the intellectual excitement which is desirable to maintain as a characteristic feature of the environment.

Of primary importance in keeping the research organization intellectually fertile is the climate of freedom. Freedom is the priceless possession of the scientist—freedom to pursue his own interests and curiosity, to make his own affiliations, to advance his program according to his own style. Even freedom to regulate the ratio of his thinking to his doing; in other words, freedom to ruminate, to daydream, to speculate, to build thought structure.

Some administrators are troubled by this freedom because it implies two worlds within the hospital universe. One is the world of practical service wherein personnel work hard, try to handle an overload of sick patients, are constantly concerned with tangible problems, and have little time for reflection. The other world is that of the scientists, who come and go as they like and are often found in their offices reading books, toying with charts, or just "thinking." The hard-working service people, too, may look upon the researchers as impractical, unproductive dreamers, who use the research life as a way of escaping from reality. It is difficult for some of them to understand why the researchers should command so much time and money.

How much time, energy, and money are in fact wasted or

poorly invested will depend in part on the administrator. The wise administrator will choose those researchers who are dedicated, inspired, and motivated, and eliminate those who in the long run are not making a contribution or who utilize the research opportunity as an escape. A motivated worker will be making advances and grow as an expert in his field visibly from month to month and year to year, and it is not difficult in the majority of cases to distinguish between a solid performer and a "loser." Also, there is usually little reason to be concerned about so-called idle periods. The average investigator puts in a great deal of time on his work. Often, in huge spurts of energy and excitement, many researchers will work around the clock. What is more, they often take on added tasks by assuming clinical responsibility for those patients who come within their research interest.

Freedom to think and work in his own way also implies for the research worker freedom to travel to other centers to inform himself of their work, to meet colleagues in the same field, to go to conferences, or to foundations and granting agencies for the sake of raising funds. Whether this travel is national or international, in our opinion it is almost always justified. Many administrators, however, are concerned that these trips represent pure junkets, despite the fact that there is usually a practical limit on travel imposed by the shortage of funds. This is especially true when funds stem mainly from state sources. However, even if travel funds were unlimited, we are convinced that travel privileges would rarely be abused. A conscientious investigator usually resents the hours spent away from the workbench; if he does not, he is one whom the research administrator will eventually direct to other pastures.

Another requirement for the researcher is the feeling that he will receive continuous and steadfast support from administration. The top administrator has to make it decisively clear that he not only values investigators highly but that he also intends to create a proper climate for their development. This support will have to be proved in the provision of space for their work, supplies, and equipment, and in administrative attention to a host of details as the investigators' frontiers unfold. At Boston State, for example, space for the first group of workers was provided in the administration building, giving them easy access to the superintendent—both formally and informally—whenever needed and without delay. Over time and as the research organization developed, new researchers needed even less special consideration and effort than the early pioneers.

Even more important support is that related to the substance and motif of the researchers' work. To be understood, to have long chats with senior people about their ideas, to observe that their major administrative figure is as excited as they are about the investigation, the challenge, and the promise: these are often the most significant ingredients for an unfolding career which at its best is fraught with stresses and frustrations, and at its worst is a long-shot effort to add something significant to the sum of human knowledge and to make a reputation doing so. I think many a young man came to feel that he was living the kind of career that I personally had lived for many years, and that I wanted to relive it with him again—the struggles, hopes, and thrills of finding out something new.

In the elaboration of a research design, in the prosecution of goals, and especially in the intensive study and editorial help with his first manuscript, the administrator, or research director, is being tested by the young worker. Is this the man from whom I can learn? Is this the man whose thought processes stimulate and inspire my own? This is what the young researcher wants to know. In order to fulfill such challenging expectations, the administrator or research director has to work at it. He has to work for the researcher and, mark this, with no thought of return, for the major requirement of a good research climate is generosity. This should spring from and be sustained by senior figures. Remember that many young people with bright vision and high drive are often very jealous of their thinking and work, and suspicious of the motives of others.

Thus, the research director has to make some very demanding requirements of himself if he expects to gain the confidence of his young workers. The first is that he too must be engaged in creative activity at some level in order to retain the respect of his colleagues and to remain in touch with some specific field in which he is attempting to achieve or maintain expertise. Active investigators are quick to know who is in the fray, who is a spectator, and who is virtually a retired general in the field. They gravitate toward senior men of experience and stature provided that the latter stay in the field. If they slacken off for a year or two, it soon becomes apparent that "the boss" has become rusty or has lost his spark. It has been said that research is a jealous mistress and a tough taskmaster; it should also be said that research workers quickly expel from their club whoever slackens seriously in his drive to create.

A strategically important point in the development of a relationship with a young worker is his first manuscript. As a matter of fact, I continually made it a rule to read not only the first draft, but most if not all of the subsequent revisions as well. Background for an understanding of the work was laid by studying any previous significant writings the researcher did, whether a thesis, collaborative article, or even raw notes. Then in a spirit of critical, objective, and sympathetic attention to his writing, editorial recommendations were made based on a hard reading and analysis of every detail. If one has had experience with research writing and editing, one can be of enormous help to the young author and make a very solid friendship besides.

Beyond the support the researcher gets in his own organization, he needs the recognition from, and affiliation with, some university or academic center. A lonely biochemist, for instance, may find it trying to be separated from his academic group, no matter how well he is set up in a hospital laboratory. Therefore, joint appointment to a relevant university department should be the rule, with plenty of latitude to join in its activities—indeed, to be considered a full-fledged member of that department. The best formula is not only joint appointment but also joint contribution to salary, and agreement by both sponsoring agencies as to the general conditions and guidelines most suitable to the research worker's continued growth and development. Evidence that the investigator is worthy of academic title is indicated not only in the university appointment and commitment to salary, but also in the opportunity to teach and to recruit students he needs to work with him. In this way, the hospital researcher keeps his laboratory at the hospital up on the latest academic developments in his field and, in return, enriches the university department from his evolving experience in the hospital environment, with its special problems and challenges.

University connections, a stimulating environment that offers sufficient freedom of thought, highly respected companionship, strong administrative support from someone who has the good will of the research group at heart, all help to compensate for what is often difficult to obtain in the mental hospital—proper space and equipment. I have seen young men who were so delighted with the opportunity to be with a stimulating group that they have been willing to pursue their work in tight and meager quarters, and even to wrestle with elaborate problems pertaining to getting their own equipment. Wherever a vigorous research department operates, it is likely that space will be at a premium; where space is not a problem, it is likely that not much research is going on. Research in the last analysis is an expansionist business, basically competitive, and often flourishes best when people are squeezed into a limited area, working elbow to elbow.

Nevertheless, there are certain minimal requirements—an office with a secretary, conference and lounge rooms, a library, a lecture hall, and, of course, equipment suitable for the specialty of the particular research worker. Laboratories with sinks, refrigerators, cold rooms, microbalances, animal rooms, and the enormously specialized apparatus of the modern scientist are very expensive, but are now the required underpinnings for basic studies in human or animal behavior, which in turn are the necessary complementaries of studies in psychology, group behavior, sociology, and so on.

Far from least in the list of requirements for the career investigator is an adequate salary. For too many years, research-minded psychiatrists were expected to pursue their activities on their own time and their own expense. Although, in our more recent past, their value on the marketplace has gone up, their salaries have been considerably lower than those earned by other professionals with comparable training. Owing largely to the efforts of the National Institute of Mental Health, career development awards have been established to encourage gifted young workers to enter the field of research. Even with such awards, however, any private practice for gain is prohibited (presumably for fear that the worker will not tend to his research); hence, a career in science is still compensated at lower levels than clinical practice. Nevertheless, the NIMH stipends and some university salaries for career researchers do recognize the unique value of the creative mind. Policy makers in government and those responsible for handling large sums of money in the public welfare at last are championing the importance of large investments in our future through adequate support of our exceptional people. These people are altogether too few in the world to be wasted.

The Young Worker

In the preceding, we have concentrated on the care and feeding of the committed researcher. But what is the approach toward those not yet committed—the young staff members or psychiatric residents who are just flirting with the idea of research? Or perhaps have even taken a few tentative steps in the direction of a research career?

Years of delightful experience living and working with bright, young psychiatric residents taught us many things. We learned that at this time in their lives, when they are preoccupied with the subtleties of therapeutic relationships, with fantasy life, with becoming emotionally attuned to the deeper feelings of patients and themselves, and trying to unravel the links between psychodynamics, sociodynamics, and biological factors, they find it difficult to embrace a research orientation with its emphasis on precision of variables, rigorous thinking and, often, to their minds, straitjacket methodological design.

Here the task of the administrator is to show them that research, in a sense, can be where the heart is. There is a methodology appropriate to every question and suitable to many styles. Having thrown off the shackles of physical-science methodology and arrived with a sigh of relief at the gates of direct human service and the study of the soul, they do not have to return completely to their former constraints. They should be shown that there are virtues and possibilities in participant and nonparticipant observation, in the use of interview techniques, and in the naturalistic style.

The second task of the administrator is to make capital out of some central problems and themes of psychiatry that are also compatible with basic principles of research: the importance of self-awareness and self-criticism, the effect of the experimenter on the subject, the concept of set, and the subtleties of interfering phenomena, such as the placebo effect. If common ground can be established, the young psychiatrist may not only be able to introduce a research approach to his special problems in clinical dynamics, but he will also take a more critical attitude toward what he is doing day by day in the care and treatment of patients.

As we worked with these young men and women we began to see that most of them were endowed with very considerable curiosity and a wholesome respect for the accomplishments of science. For many, however, there were blocks, impasses, or resistances that prevented them from applying their professionally valued curiosity systematically to some research area. The resistances were really of the same nature as defense mechanisms, similar in structure and development to the ordinary psychopathologies of everyday life that we all possess. If they could be freed of these emotional obstacles they could move further along the road to wholesome, enjoyable, and even distinguished indulgence of their natural curiosity drive.

These resistances fell into several types. Some who had been involved in research before their resident-training had been doing work in the basic sciences: animal research, biochemistry, and the like, where highly meticulous methodology had been applied.

Their loyalty was to that field of research, not to psychiatry. They often felt that the techniques mastered in other fields were totally inapplicable to psychiatry—an erroneous judgment. Others suffered from what one would describe as an overcritical research superego. They would not undertake anything unless it finished "perfect." They held a low opinion of most of the research done in psychiatry: "The journals are full of trash. . . . There is a lot of publishing for publication's sake." "True progress is the work of a few geniuses; all the rest is negligible." Sometimes they gave the impression that they were impatient with having to begin with a small project and subject themselves to the disciplines of a narrow methodology. They were waiting for the blinding insight, the real big idea that would change everything. Negative identifications typified still another orientation. One young staff member had an uncle who was a brilliant research microbiologist. He admired his knowledge, the clarity of his thinking, the purity of his experimental design, and the preciseness of his findings, but he did not like his uncle. He also vented considerable resentment against a number of prominent figures in the research firmament; they tended to publish too much and they strove too hard for prestige and academic attainment.

It is possible for such blocks to be dealt with in the same manner as any other personality problem. But as a first step, everyone who comes to the administrator to discuss his interests should be given aid and encouragement. The attitude should be that few ideas are really bad and that most ideas can be evolved into better concepts, if intelligently discussed. Moreover, every worker should be encouraged not only for that which he begins today, but also for that which he may be able to do in the years ahead.

Grantsmanship

The young researcher may think he is all set when he gets his own laboratory, his university affiliation, his equipment, his salary, his secretary, and his assistant. Initially he has fantasies of "staying small." "Bigness" would transform him into an administrator, who has to be concerned with budget, hiring and firing, personnel problems, and so on. He is properly concerned with freeing as much of his time as possible for creative work, and wonders what is the smallest possible unit he can manage in order to insure his maximum personal productivity over a long time.

But the numerous, inescapable details of supervision of any project, no matter how minute, make deep inroads into his time and attention. Furthermore, there is the inevitable search for funds. Few universities or hospitals can guarantee sufficient funds from their hard-money income to look after the growing needs of an active, successful researcher. The investigator of today almost regularly, sooner or later, becomes a supplicant before foundations and granting agencies. Altogether reluctantly, he is soon in the business of fund-raising and as such he is in competition with many, many other workers and with some who have made a specialty of grant-getting.

Although much of this must have been obvious from the beginning of his career, the young researcher is nevertheless a bit shaken when his administrator reminds him that additional funds, even for a secretary, another trip afield, or a minor structural renovation in his department are not immediately available but that the money has to be raised afresh. It is at this point that the administrator must initiate the young scientist into the hard realities of fiscal management and begin to teach him the art of raising money for research, a detail that may have been omitted from his previous training.

However noxious the task may appear to him in the beginning, the investigator must of necessity learn the discipline required in raising funds. First, he has to think precisely about what he is doing and where he is going, formulate his problem in exact language, and then relate his interest to the *raison d'être* of the granting agency or foundation. Foundations all have their specific roles, their own concepts of how they can best serve the public. They are also sometimes interested in what the research they support may do to their public image and their own good name.

Almost inevitably, fund-raising means making the acquaintance of individuals representing granting agencies and foundations at the executive level. This must be done early, with a lead time of at least two years before the request for support is to be made. Also, there is the necessity to study backgrounds, credentials, and probably voting records of members of advisory committees, study groups, or decision-making bodies, by whatever name they are called. The young researcher must pay a good deal of attention not only to the precision of his aims, the appropriateness of his methods, the probability of arriving at an answer to significant questions within a finite period of time (three to five years), but he must also present in fullest array the potentiality of his research for improving the lot of man.

The young investigator not only needs help in the preparation of his application, in negotiating with granting agencies, and in presenting his case before critical colleagues, but—and this is even more important—he also needs support and encouragement by the administrator to tide him over the inevitable disappointments. If he stays in research long enough, he will have more than a few applications turned down, but this is especially painful in the early years of his career. Not a few aspiring young investigators have thrown in the sponge altogether after one or two early rejections and have left the field. It can be a terrible blow to their morale and their research ego. Therefore, the administrator or research director should prepare the individual beforehand for the possibility of a rejection and, if there is one, support him until his hope and enthusiasm return. He should be told never to assume that the negative judgment of a board of reviewers, no matter how distinguished they may be, is necessarily a true measure of his worth as a researcher.

But whatever the judgment of the foundation or granting agency, it is good to establish a policy of requesting the board's critique in detail, for there is usually much to learn from their evaluation. A reapplication that integrates recommendations and suggestions made by this body is often successful where the first may have failed.

Fund-raising is often as demanding of skill, energy, and creative thinking as the research itself. One of the hardest adjustments upon learning what the trends and interest of granting agencies may be is to rethink one's project in the light of what will fit best with that agency's interests and in a sense further its goals. The young idealistic researcher may see this as a prostitution of his career and may object violently on principle. But oddly enough, this is where he has to learn the most. He has to face the realities of life and not live in a fantasy world. At certain times and certain places, a certain kind of research endeavor is rewarded. There are fads and fashions in this field as in so many others.

This is a hard pill to swallow, but several considerations may soften the blow. First is the understanding that so-called fads and fashions in research are usually based on considerable study and deep thought given by the foundations as to the needs of humanity. Second is the fact that often quite minor modifications of goal or methods, or even phraseology, may make it possible for a foundation to look with favor on a project as now within its frame of reference, although it had been rejected before. The third is insight that one's skill as a *researcher in the generalized sense* is greatly needed, even though the pursuit of one's specific interests may sometimes have to be postponed. It may not be possible to follow one's greatest curiosity and interest every moment in time. Compromises may have to be made here as elsewhere. It is best not to be too rigid and sacrifice a life of scientific productivity simply because the urge of the moment has been temporarily blocked.

The young investigator who is blessed with a certain amount of innate wisdom realizes that, during his lifetime, both he and his research will change, often influenced by subtle and largely unconscious factors, such as a chance meeting with a stimulating colleague or another way of looking at his own data. He can then accept more readily the fact that he may have to change also in relation to external pressures, such as foundation policies—usually open, explicit, and quite rational. Too, in many cases, he may be able to choose among a number of foundations that support his field, selecting the one most appropriate to his trends. And in all this, again, the administrator may be of help to him since some of his problem of adaptation may be due to inexperience or naïveté. In some special cases, judgment will dictate that the young researcher should be left strictly alone to work out his problem in his own way.

It should not be assumed that the administrator can act merely as a grant-application consultant or advisor. Rather, it is necessary that he also join seriously in the search for funds because the usual grant bestowed upon individual investigators leaves very little or no room for fiscal flexibility. If funds are needed to hire another librarian, to make a feasibility study of biostatistical technology, to renovate a building for expansion, or to do anything outside the range of a specific project, he must find a way to raise that money. This he must do through the same kind of hard work that he has been expecting from his subordinates.

Finally, a word about the hard money–soft money ratio. Years ago research was almost entirely under the university roof; money was tight, but was essentially hard money—that is, securely based on fixed, usually endowment, income. Today, the universities, the hospitals, and most private research organizations depend to a great extent on soft money—that is, short-term support raised from federal agencies, foundations, and corporations. A few, but only a few, establishments have refused to join this soft-money trend of recent years and have depended primarily on state support; the vast majority are drinking at the federal troughs or the fountains of private foundations.

It goes almost without saying that every effort should be made to establish research on the most solid long-term basis possible, and both federal (before Vietnam) and private foundations have shown a considerable tendency to give long-term support. The development of research career awards previously mentioned is but one example. However, after many years of steady growth in federal expenditures for research in all fields, and especially in mental health, unanticipated and dramatic reductions can suddenly occur, as a result of other pressures for federal monies, as Vietnam well reminds us. To guard against retrenchments of this sort, great efforts must be expended to educate state and local agencies to assume responsibility for crisis periods, not to mention continuing basic aid for long periods and at substantial levels.

Research as an Instrument for Social and Organizational Change

The power of research as an instrument for social and organizational change is often insufficiently recognized. It is especially effective when change is resisted by a rigid, entrenched hierarchy or is dependent on state funds, difficult to obtain and often highly restricted in use, or when change depends on developing new values or changing old ones. Here one finds that the research approach can be a flexible tool for cracking old ways of thinking, for introducing pilot demonstrations, for intellectualizing, conceptualizing, and objectifying that which has become routine, entrenched, and unquestioned. Therefore, the early development of a research component that bears directly on issues of institutional change is essential. Among the numerous advantages, there are three that are worth underscoring:

1. Research on issues of direct patient care and hospital organization is closer to the interests of clinical staff than are basic laboratory investigations In some instances, they will be moved to participate in such studies themselves. In many more, they will be stimulated in their own work by having research going on around them. There is likely to be less resentment from clinical people toward research that bears directly on their concerns than that whose practical implications may not be clear for a long time.

2. The state hospital is rich in examples of organizational as well as individual pathology. If the administrator supports research in this area, a special group of investigators highly significant in the elucidation of organizational dynamics will be drawn to the state setting.

3. Through social and organizational research, the administrator's commitment to change can be intellectually enriched and often practically furthered.

We will cite a few brief examples of research studies at Boston

State which bore directly on issues of patient care and overall hospital policy.

A grant for training residents made it possible to recruit an investigator interested in the process of education for all personnel trained at the hospital. As described in the previous chapter, his survey of residents' needs, complaints, and special interests led to a thorough reorganization of the training program. His studies showed us that the home treatment service was considered to be of high teaching value to residents, but that experience in the chronic services was unrewarding. Much effort subsequently went into bringing chronic services in line with the training programs in other parts of the hospital.

The study of nursing homes generated sufficient interest among staff in geriatric illness to spill over into their clinical work with the elderly. Moreover, the research data showed that patients sent to nursing homes by Boston State were as well behaved as those patients referred from medical hospitals and that the latter, contrary to the popular stereotypes, also demonstrated a high incidence of mental disturbances. This finding was often used as an argument with proprietors of nursing homes who might be prejudiced against accepting patients directly from mental hospitals, even those who were especially selected for their good psychological status. The investigation also showed that, in contrast to a control group, nursing homes that were provided with consultation and instruction for their problems by the Boston State geriatric research team fared much better with their patients and, more than incidentally, had a much lower death rate.[13]

The psychopharmacologist mentioned previously set up an office of drug research which, over the course of time, introduced the teaching of drug therapy to residents and staff and reorganized the program of drug administration. One of his associates took over the management of an entire building of one hundred chronic patients and pursued vigorously a treatment program that combined drug therapy and work rehabilitation.[14] In time most of his patients were discharged so that with concomitant population reductions in other parts of the hospital, it was possible to absorb his unit into another building. This, fortunately, meant a consolidation of staffs, a higher personnel-patient ratio, and a further intensification of individualized treatment.

Two social workers undertook an important study on the use of volunteers as case aides,[15] which eventually led to several grants for further research in that area and a broadening of community involvement within the hospital. Well over a hundred volunteers were paired with chronic patients who through the efforts of the volunteers learned to take greater advantage of the hospital's programs and gradually to negotiate the move back into the life of the community. The volunteers were directly responsible for the community resettling of hundreds of patients, and by their continued interest stimulated the development of bridging programs. Talented volunteers, after a year or more experience under social work guidance, themselves began to train other volunteers in the art of "friendship therapy" on a one-to-one basis —thus accomplishing an ultimate extension of the clinical effectiveness of supervision. The value to the volunteer of these experiences was considerable, and the value to the hospital of involved and experienced volunteers functioning as quasi-public relations officers in the community was inestimable. Their success in that investigation and others, including the one on adolescents (chapter 5), helped legitimate research as a branch of social work, a discipline that had previously been chiefly service oriented.

In an effort to explore as many facets of our therapeutic organization as possible, we especially sought out students in social psychology and social science from local universities and invited their research not only on patient care but on institutional change as well. The studies ranged from hard-nosed fact-finding investigations to perceptive human documents written by students who may have lacked methodological refinement but who were rich in their penetrating insights into human suffering and indignity. Sometimes, the shock of seeing ourselves as others saw us was almost more than we could stand, and the tendency to deny or cover up was almost irresistible. Needless to say, however, we expended great efforts in finding ways to utilize the reports in a positive and constructive fashion.

In the interest of brevity and readability, we have chosen one such report for examination, taking at times some liberties in presenting the findings.[16] The study takes on added significance when the reader bears in mind that it is the work of a youthful investigator, one of the many young people who were encouraged to conduct the kind of research that added to the hospital's growth as fully as it did to their own.

This young man, a medical student at Tufts, interviewed patients on their second day of hospitalization to ascertain their reaction to the process of admission and to validate impressions from direct observation of that procedure. He found that most often patients were brought not to the front entrance of the admissions unit, but to the side door, or to a shabby rear entrance opposite the garbage pile and incinerator. Once inside, they might wait three to four hours before seeing a doctor or an attendant. Meanwhile, they were ignored by all and spent most of their time wandering aimlessly up and down the corridors or sitting silently on old uncomfortable chairs, without anything to read, listening to typewriters and secretaries in adjacent offices. The possibility that this waiting period could aggravate anxieties or fearful fantasies was not of apparent concern to the staff.

When the admitting physician finally appeared, he interviewed the patients in a bleak, shabbily furnished room. They were then taken to another room to be weighed and then to be given a physical examination, separated from other patients by only an insecurely closed curtain, an arrangement affording little privacy.

Staff attitudes, according to the observer, reflected condescension, lack of concern, and an apparent view of the patients as children or incompetents.

Explanations were not given as to why keys, jewelry, and money were taken away, or why the patient was to go to the ward, or what kind of ward to expect. When taken to the ward, the new patient often confronted blank faces: he was not introduced to the other patients, nor was he given a tour of the ward, or any orientation as to facilities for living and recreation.

The report, apart from its exposure of gross deficiencies in the admission procedure, called attention to a deeper problem. During the years that the hospital population had been declining, especially on the overcrowded chronic services, a concomitant and opposite rise in admissions had taken place, straining increasingly the ability of the admission team to process cases, and finally leading to a serious overload. The admission procedure became hurried; almost imperceptibly staff's interest in making the patient's first contact humane and therapeutic slipped out of focus and callous attitudes took over. It was not until a sensitive and objective person reported his findings that the hospital was shocked into reality.

The first corrective measure was to make the report widely known and to indicate that admission was a vital and continuing concern of administration. The second was to emphasize the need for careful supervision of the admission procedure by the most experienced personnel, and not to leave this process entirely in the hands of first-year residents or untrained nurses.

The third plan was to extend and intensify the functions of a newly developed screening service to include a larger number of patients. The eight-bed screening service had evolved in 1963 as one means of combatting both the overload and the routinization of admissions. By giving intensive attention over a period of one to five days to a selected 25 percent of all admissions, the service had been able to return about 80 percent of those patients to the community. The screening team utilized the day hospital, outpatient department, and community resources much more actively than did the regular admission service. The expanded screening service was then moved out of the reception building, where it was first established, to more spacious quarters in a newly constructed community-services building and placed under the jurisdiction of the outpatient department.

A fourth measure was to unitize the hospital into decentralized services, each with its own admission ward, so that the heavy load of admissions was spread throughout the four units. With a smaller load, each unit could concentrate more on the individual needs of the newly admitted patients, with special concern to avoid the degrading and dehumanizing procedures pointed out by the report.

Thus, one research study acted as an instrument to stimulate changes in certain hospital practices that had been dysfunctional to the system as a whole.

The Researcher as a Teacher

Another way in which the research organization can serve as an instrument for institutional change is in teaching. It should accept as one of its functions the enhancement of the curiosity and the interest of everyone in the system. It should also assume that many are able to contribute who are now restrained by pressures of routine or by lack of recognition or stimulation of their innate creative abilities. Sooner or later, the core research people must impart to others the fact that they too have ideas and suggestions that are vital to the expansion of their roles and to patient care and that there are methods appropriate to their stage of development that can be utilized to structure their search for knowledge.

Once again, it should be emphasized that if these clinical people possess an advanced academic degree it may be a help, but lack of it should not be a reason for exclusion. The highly trained research specialist should not be too critical of, or impatient with, the efforts of "untrained" staff to find ways to improve their role through self-study. For if personnel at the ward level do not give attention to the solution of their own problems, it may be a long time indeed before highly trained persons will come to their rescue. Researchers tend to become entranced with the more theoretical, esoteric aspects of problems relating to patient care, with little payoff to the individual who wants to know in a practical way—and right now—how to do his job better.

Since experimental programs do not run at high pitch all the time, but often go by fits and starts, the researcher should be available during these quiet periods to act in a teaching role. Moreover, we have found that even though the researcher jealously guards his privacy, he also finds it stimulating to be part of the hospital activities, to rub elbows with individuals who might be in the training or service division and often to collaborate with them.

The researcher should be given the responsibility to report progress on his work at intervals to the general staff and to give instruction to various groups in the area of his growing expertise. A necessary condition for the teaching function of researchers, however, is a well-developed educational system and the integration of research with training programs of staff at all levels. Given this communication with different divisions of the hospital, not only can a group of professionals who specifically chose research as a career be trained, but also people of all disciplines can be taught how to undertake studies suited to their levels of interest and skill. Thus a special climate will pervade the whole institution, namely, more intellectual effort, more interest in new demonstrations, a sense of criticism, an alertness to new ways of looking at things, a greater appreciation of talent and imagination possessed by others.

Summary

We have said more than enough to indicate our conviction that the development of a research department—and in particular the cultivation of the research atmosphere—is a sine qua non in the rehabilitation of a large mental hospital. Research is a formal way of looking at ourselves, our roles, our values, our results; it demands rigor and disciplined thinking; it is a tool for social action and generates important institutional change; it is a link to the academic community, the community of scholars, and those who search for excellence; it is a feature that attracts talented men and women to the hospital and helps recruitment at all levels; it is a function that attracts funds; it imparts a special premium to ideas, to inspiration, and to new ways of looking at things.

But research must be sparked by dedicated research workers. On the present scene, there are relatively few committed researchers, and with the recent diminution of available funds, there may be fewer in the future. The young man (or woman) who is ready to embark on a professional career must still give up a great deal if he chooses to become a researcher—clinical practice, the opportunity to earn enough money for relative affluence, and a life free of the rigors of experimentation and sharp collegial criticism.

The mental hospital needs these researchers as a part of its total development. Although the task of building a research organization in a hospital outside of, and at some distance from, the university establishment is great, that task can be immeasurably lightened if the hospital administrator has had research training, has established a reputation in some field, has upheld the research philosophy, and is himself currently engaged in creative activity.

REFERENCES

1. E. Hartmann, *The Biology of Dreaming* (Springfield, Ill.: Charles C Thomas, 1967).

2. B. Stotsky, *The Elderly Patient: Mental Patients in Nursing Homes* (New York: Grune and Stratton, 1968).

3. D. Kantor and V. A. Gelineau, "Making Chronic Schizophrenics," *Mental Hygiene* 53, no. 1 (1969): 54–66.

4. T. McLardy, "Thalamic Microneurones," *Nature* 199 (1963): 820–21, and "Fornix Function During Behavior Formative Age," *Scientific Proceedings of the American Psychiatric Association* 124 (1968): 42–43.

5. A. DiMascio and J. M. Levine, "A Step Toward Prediction of Clinical Efficacy: Relationship of History and Initial Characteristics of Patients to Improvement," in *Drug and Social Therapy in Chronic Schizophrenia*, ed. M. Greenblatt et al. (Springfield, Ill.: Charles C Thomas, 1965).

6. J. Arsenian and E. V. Semrad, " 'Depth' Levels in Individual Group Manifestations," *International Journal of Group Psychotherapy* 27 (1967): 82–97.

7. M. R. Sharaf and D. J. Levinson, "Patterns of Ideology and Role Definition Among Psychiatric Residents," in *The Patient and the Mental Hospital*, ed. M. Greenblatt, D. J. Levinson, and R. H. Williams (Glencoe: Free Press, 1957), pp. 263–85; J. Kotin and M. R. Sharaf, "Intrastaff Con-

troversy at a State Mental Hospital: An Analysis of Ideological Issues," *Psychiatry* 30 (1967): 16–29; Kotin and Sharaf, "Management Succession and Administrative Style," ibid., pp. 237–48; M. R. Sharaf and M. Greenblatt, "Attitudes of Psychiatric Residents Toward Milieu Therapy," *Social Psychiatry* 9 (1968): 142–56.

8. H. C. Schulberg and F. Baker, "The Changing Mental Hospital: A Progress Report," *Hospital and Community Psychiatry* 20 (1969): 159–65.

9. D. C. Gilbert and D. J. Levinson, " 'Custodialism' and 'Humanism' in Mental Hospital Structure and in Staff Ideology," in *The Patient and the Mental Hospital*, pp. 20–35; and E. B. Gallagher, D. J. Levinson, and I. Erlich, "Some Socio-psychological Characteristics of Patients and Their Relevance for Psychiatric Treatment," in ibid., pp. 357–79.

10. L. Weiner, "Developing a Consultation Program for Primary Physicians at a State Hospital," *Frontiers of Hospital Psychiatry*, Roche Report 5, no. 3 (February 1968).

11. L. Weiner et al., *Home Treatment: Spearhead of Community Psychiatry* (Pittsburgh: University of Pittsburgh Press, 1967); Stotsky, *The Elderly Patient*; Hartmann, *Biology*; A. Becker, ed., *The General Practitioner's Role in the Treatment of Emotional Illness* (Springfield, Ill.: Charles C Thomas, 1968); and E. Hartmann et al., eds., *Adolescents in a Mental Hospital* (New York: Grune and Stratton, 1968).

12. F. P. Gay, *The Open Mind: Elmer Ernest Southard* (Chicago: Normandie House, 1938).

13. Stotsky, *The Elderly Patient*.

14. Ching-piao Chien, "Some Factors Deciding the Discharge of Chronic Mental Patients," *Hospital and Community Psychiatry* (in press).

15. V. A. Celineau and A. Evans, "Volunteer Case Aides Rehabilitate Chronic Patients," *Hospital and Community Psychiatry* 21 (1970): 90–93.

16. F. Coplon, "The First Twenty-Four Hours at Boston State Hospital," unpublished data.

Epilogue

By Milton Greenblatt

As this book goes to press, I have the advantage of more than three years out of the office of superintendent. The opportunity is to look back, to reflect on what we have learned, its bearing on career development, what such experience could mean for other psychiatrists making decisions about their future; above all, what the relatively brief four-year term as hospital administrator may have meant to the institution in the pursuit of its own goals.

My vantage point is a broad one, for I became commissioner of mental health for Massachusetts immediately upon leaving the hospital. As commissioner, I have Boston State as one of my responsibilities. Immediately the question arises whether, from the new viewpoint, the innovations developed in the four-year tenure are worth continuing; also, of course, whether the philosophies of institutional change at Boston State could be generalized through all hospitals under state and government aegis.

We found it relevant and reasonable to call for statewide application of what was learned at Boston State; for example, unitization, work rehabilitation, adolescent and home treatment services, wider use of volunteers, the solidifying of relationships with community clinics, a more flexible use of personnel. Many of the hospitals had already made excellent strides in these directions and, indeed, some had preceded Boston State years before in specific endeavors and accomplishments. One, for example, was using nurses in roles formerly entirely preempted by social workers in order to help the process of discharge of patients and reduction of census. Another was one of the earlier experimenters in unitization; and another pioneered greatly in work rehabilitation. All have continued in their movement toward reduction of inpatient census by improved community care. For example, the population at Boston State, under the imaginative and dynamic leadership of my successor, Jonathan Cole, is now down to a little more than nine hundred patients.

Two impressions are carried both from the job as hospital administrator and as commissioner: one is the extraordinary need for persons to occupy leadership posts in the new community and comprehensive health care era; the other is the extraordinary scarcity of individuals interested in taking leadership jobs or enthusiastic about their potentialities.

The new community health system of America cannot be built in a leadership vacuum. The vast multiplication of facilities, the explosion of new concepts in models of delivery of care, the integration of hospital with community, the expansion of total health care to include systems like mental illness, retardation, alcoholism and drug addiction, welfare, crime, delinquency, the enlargement of social-environmental concepts to embrace the whole ecosystem of man—all these sharpen the need for leaders in a period of veritable revolutionary change in service. For better or worse, there is evolving an ultimate goal of a guarantee of adequate and appropriate services for all. It is clear that the Constitution's guarantee of life, liberty, and pursuit of happiness is being interpreted in our modern age to include the right of health. The courts are producing opinions declaring the right of adequate treatment, and new mental health legislation in some of the states incorporates this. Above all, the average citizen knows instinctively that life is a poor gift without health; liberty cannot mean much unless one is free from crippling disease; and happiness depends upon having a sound mind and body.

In the face of sharply expanding expectations, trained manpower lags far behind; and able, creative administration seems to be the primary need everywhere. In the field of health, we rarely have consciously trained executives in the same way that we have trained psychotherapists, surgeons, internists, and the like. We have expected a vast army of professional caregivers to fill individual human needs, mainly on a laissez-faire basis, mostly without planning, without coordination, without sufficient concern for lost Americans, who either do not look for care, cannot afford it, or cannot get to it.

With little or no formal training, administrators—particularly in the field of mental health—have arisen from our midst willy-nilly, too few through natural ability, too many by virtue of their staying power on a particular job, lack of available competition, or the administrator's uncritical need for power and control. Little dignity, status, or academic distinction often accompanies the role. No exciting ideology pervades its functions. In industry, by contrast, there is far more recognition and reward for the role of the administrator, for profits and competition have raised his function to a critical significance. Proportionately much thought, writing and training have gone into explication and development of the executive role in business management. In mental health administration, on the other hand, there are few theoreticians, few training centers, few books, and an almost absolute dearth of strict scientific investigations.

Nowhere is this more apparent than in the large state hospital system, which, to a great extent, is being overshadowed in significance by recent emphasis on comprehensive community health centers and community care. Furthermore, the strain of management in the large hospital is exaggerated by lack of manpower resources, by inadequate financing, and excessive numbers of severely ill patients. Thus, where the needs are greatest, and the difficulties of management most burdensome, the chances of success depend mightily on the energy and resourcefulness of the executive figure.

A large therapeutic organization such as a mental hospital serves many masters: patients, families, staff, community, legislators, the department of mental health, and the governor. There are many watchdogs and many critics, both within the hospital and outside its walls. Since the commodity it produces, mental health, is precious, difficult to define, and difficult to produce, a great deal of misinterpretation and emotionalism accompanies its manufacture. Added to this is the fact that the product must be turned out under conditions of massive overload, major manpower shortage, and serious physical and social impoverishment. Under these conditions management, particularly the top administrator, is exceedingly vulnerable. Partly as a protective device and primarily as a means of producing better patient care and treatment, it behooves management to be inordinately self-critical. The best place to begin is with oneself, and from my own experience, the first critical phase I have often reviewed in my mind is management succession.

Management succession is a dramatic and disturbing event in almost all organizations; only a few have been left unscathed by the impact of the new man coming in with new ideas, vigorous and eager to make his mark. Most of us appreciate from our own experience the turmoil, unrest, and insecurity produced by a change in top command. Indeed, many large institutions have a tradition of mass resignations when the new chief takes over. This is partly to anticipate the dreaded firing that may occur as the "new broom sweeps clean," partly to give the new man a free hand. Historically, one result of this threat to job security has been the increased emphasis in our bureaucratic systems on tenure and civil service benefits. Yet, even when the objective risks of losing one's job are minimal, and the new administrator is known to bring only himself and no band of cronies, the disturbance in the organization can be profound.

Before the successor is acknowledged as the new leader, the organization often goes through several stages in the process of acceptance. The first is the anticipatory anxiety over his arrival. There is much gossip about him. He is often painted as tough and ruthless, a man who makes hard decisions without the kind indulgences to human frailities that categorized his predecessor. The old boss is idealized, and a common refrain is: "We will never have it so good again." This feeling prevails particularly where the departing commander has been around a long time and has built up a stable and efficient team whose work has been crowned with success and recognition. And even for those who see in the succession new opportunities for acceptance and advancement, the future is still viewed with uneasiness, and anxiety pervades the organization.

The second stage occurs when the new administrator arrives. Surprisingly, he is a human being and not an ogre. He seems to want to be liked. He smiles generously and pays attention, and he genuinely cares about achieving acceptance from personnel and advancing the true goals of the organization. There is an institutional sigh of relief and the honeymoon begins.

After the honeymoon comes the third stage in which employees begin to miss the familiar, the support and security of accustomed practices. They test out the new leader in a variety of ways, from having heart-to-heart talks with him about their work and their futures, to bringing in complaints, and making demands for change. Some suddenly discover they know a great deal more about their job than they thought, and are in a position to teach the incumbent, who may know far less in the particular area than the former chief. The new man is constantly and mercilessly compared with the old. As his program unfolds, decisions are made which some believe to be discriminatory against them. The new chief gathers around him a new set of advisors and those who had been *in* now feel left out. The equilibrium is upset. Supposedly unworthy people are allowed too readily into the inner sanctum. New ideology clashes with old, and people begin to think of leaving or in fact they resign. A few who are seen by the new management as not pulling their own weight, or as replaceable perhaps by persons more harmonious with the new administration, are fired or squeezed out. This phase can be a long, protracted period of trial, reorganization, and working through.

Eventually a new equilibrium is established. The tensions, differences, and clashes burn out, are openly resolved or go underground. The new man is mostly accepted for what he is, and the future depends now on his overall ability to lead, to command respect, to mobilize resources, to release creative activity, to innovate, to inspire loyalty, and to evoke effective performance from his associates.

All four phases were evident in my succession at Boston State. The former chief, the eminent Dr. Walter E. Barton, had served the hospital and served it well for seventeen years prior to my arrival. Through his efforts, what had been mainly an asylum had begun its transformation into a hospital. He was a man much honored by his profession, his dignity and integrity were highly respected, and his capacity for survival through hard times (which had beset the hospital especially early in his career) was much admired.

In this case the Rebecca myth operated well, namely, idealization of the old chief and some derogation and suspicion of the new man. This was manifest to me from reports that many members of the Boston State staff had contacted staff members of the Massachusetts Mental Health Center to inquire about my personality, my methods, and my goals. Often, it was nurse to nurse, steward to steward, social worker to social worker—each consulting his homologue in the other institution.

During the three months before my assumption of responsibility as superintendent, I was spending approximately two half days a week consulting with Dr. Barton at length, receiving orientation and instruction, interviewing heads and assistant heads of departments, as well as appearing, usually unannounced, in various buildings and wards to make my own observations. Wherever I went, I asked questions. My impression is that during this period some of the suspiciousness and anxiety was probably worked through. After I arrived on the scene in April 1963, there was a round of receptions, many interviews and discussions of how things would go in the future. Everyone was assured that his job was secure, and that I expected to study the situation in considerable detail before making any major moves. As a consequence there was a considerable relaxation of tension. It was apparent that my general goals for the institution coincided almost completely with Dr. Barton's, and in this sense there would be continuity. However, since I had not declared exactly where I would begin, or how fast I would go about it, or who exactly would be included in the executive constellation, there was still room for restiveness. Also it must have been apparent that my style would necessarily be different from Dr. Barton's and surely many must have sensed the fact of my relative ignorance of the workings of a large institution and how much I personally would have to learn.

The honeymoon period was of short duration because of the sudden need for dramatic action to meet the demands of hospital accreditation. Scarcely had we visited the fifty-odd buildings on the campus and begun to make the acquaintance of key staff members when we were informed by the Joint Commission on Accreditation of Hospitals that our inspection, formerly scheduled for November, had been moved forward to August. When our pleas for postponement were turned down, we knew we had a major crisis on our hands.

Because of two consecutive previous deferments of full accreditation, the hospital was facing a serious threat. It would be either "make" or "break." The rules of the game were that we would either have to achieve full accreditation or total disaccreditation would be our lot, with all the dire consequences of loss of status and prestige as a treatment institution, and the subsequent disaccreditation of training programs. The damage that would be done to the image of the hospital, its ability to attract able professionals, and its opportunity to achieve leadership in training and research would be almost incalculable.

A crash program was instituted. All department heads were brought together, made aware of previous criticisms and recommendations of the Joint Commission on Accreditation, charged with the task of becoming thoroughly familiar with the accreditation requirements that fell within their domain of responsibility, and told to exert every effort to see that all procedures necessary to meet accreditation criteria were done promptly and well. Management, for its part, kept up pressure for performance and checked almost daily to record progress.

Elaborate problems had to be solved, such as bringing masses of records up to date when serious shortages existed in the typing pool; handling overcrowding by more discriminating admission policy and more rapid turnover of cases; or redistributing nurses so that the required minimum of coverage could be met, especially in the acute wards, where adequate coverage was particularly emphasized by accreditation standards. All this entailed, within a narrowly circumscribed period of time, a very large educational job, exhaustive search for resources, and new organizational mechanisms for quality control.

The upshot of the accreditation crisis was that after many weeks of intensive day and night work, in which almost all hospital personnel responded with gratifying effort, many working far beyond the call of duty, the hospital finally received full accreditation, and danger was averted. The excitement of a hard-won success, and the good fellowship generated by all-out teamwork were celebrated by all the staff with an accreditation party. This was the beginning of a special understanding between the new administrator and his staff: together we had faced a serious crisis and won a significant success; the hospital had been saved by our concerted efforts from a crippling set-back. All gave unstintingly without thought of specific reward except the hospital's good. With this spirit of cooperative action, what could we not accomplish in the future?

In the successful times ahead, there were many occasions to recall our teamwork in meeting the crisis of accreditation. It was the beginning of self-confidence and the realization of our potential. Three years later, for example, having learned well how to do it, the hospital passed the next accreditation examination with flying colors.

The battle for accreditation sharpened our early awareness of the size of the job to be done, and the lack of resources at hand. We were impressed with the need to develop lieutenants to help us accomplish the task we were setting for ourselves, and to avoid further crises in the future.

Even if accreditation had not intervened, the honeymoon period would have been destined for early termination simply because the aspirations of the new leadership were so different from what the old lieutenants were used to. It was not lack of ability on their part so much as the demands of a totally different orientation and philosophy. Most were trained to give service, based as far as possible on analytic-dynamic understanding applied to psychotic patients. They had never been trained in research and development. Searching for funds, innovating programs, writing-up ideas, and peripatetic salesmanship with foundations were inimical to their self-concepts as professionals. *That* was administration's problem. Demands put on them to do these jobs would only weaken patient care. Furthermore, even where staff was more or less friendly to these concepts, they could not understand the sense of urgency. The new administration, with its dreams of activities on many fronts, wanted to find people who would carry a spirit of enterprise and urgency to all parts of the hospital. The ball was being passed to those who could scrounge, the fund raisers, the project developers, the doers, and the professionals with conventional ideas were beginning to feel left out.

The old guard responded with vigorous and outspoken defenses of their positions; there were sharp ideological clashes. Some were grimly resistive or foretold doom; others tried to learn how to meet the new expectations; most decided to sit tight. Several executives charged lack of support, meddling, or by-passing of their authority. As a matter of fact, this was true in some cases, especially if department heads were opposed to the new program or dragged their feet unduly. Since firing in a state system of civil service tenure was most difficult and resistance to change often withstood all logic and reasoning, one had little recourse but to seek creative people down the line who were willing to go ahead on the authority of the superintendent. If, as sometimes happened, this person was one who had been somewhat fractious in the past and difficult for his supervisors to control, it is not hard to understand the distress and turmoil engendered in a department when such a person got the nod. Administrative decisions of this sort are most difficult to make and extraordinarily hard for the disaffected supervisors to bear.

But, on more than one occasion, hard decisions had to be made where organizational rigidities and role protection maneuvers were depriving the institution of changes with a high promise of improving patient care and treatment.

The resignation of several department chiefs opened up opportunities to choose individuals more resonant to the new ideology. In addition, the later influx of new money made it possible to add to the staff at critical levels and to introduce new members into policy development and decision-making groups. Program development was then easier: new ideas came to the fore, many of which received reasonable trial or testing. During the two to three years in which the stresses and strains were being accommodated, management became more able and comfortable in working within the traditional authority lines which had formerly often been transcended; and department heads became more tolerant of the "loose" administrative style of the new administrator.

In a study previously mentioned,[1] Kotin and Sharaf identified a dimension of administrative style which at one end they call "tight" and at the other end "loose." Tight administrative style is characterized in the extreme as involving clear-cut delegation of authority and responsibility; orderly and hierarchical chain of command through which communication flows upward and downward without skipping levels; reliance on formal communications, for example, regular meetings, reports, printed forms; formal expression of power, for example, hearings, written notifications of promotions and dismissals; and reliance on explicit written rules or, in their absence, on tradition. Loose administrative style is characterized by absence in many areas of clearly designated authority and responsibility; considerable tolerance of role ambiguity and role diffusion; frequent by-passing of chain of command, both in communication and in authority; informal communication; informal exercise of power; relatively little reliance on rules and tradition.

This dimension could indeed prove fruitful as one way of conceptualizing administrative style, and as far as Sharaf and Kotin claim, may be highly related to the personalities of administrators.

Future research will determine how reliably administrators can be classified along this continuum. I would certainly see myself as tending toward the "loose" side of the axis, my philosophy being that "tightness" as defined above can limit flexibility and reduce creativity. Often one sees creativity linked to striving for freedom, independence and nonrestraint. These traits do not tolerate the structure of routine. To me one's administrative style would depend on how highly one values creativity.

In my experience a tight system is good for those who are comfortable with order, structure, clarity of role definition, and clear lines of authority. They are anxious under conditions of ambiguity, role-blurring, lack of control, and change, the conditions that usually release ideas, discover innovations, and create movement.

Another factor to be considered is that a tight structure often is based upon overconcern for authority and power. This was the problem in many traditional mental hospitals, which because of such emphasis failed to discover and utilize therapeutic capacities latent within many segments and echelons of the hospital community.

It should be recognized, too, that any demonstrated preference of administrative style along the tight-loose continuum does not preclude behavior that is tight in one instance and loose in another, or that is tight in one area of administration and loose in another. Obviously, if the head of a given department fails to share the administrative philosophy, is slow to learn, or temperamentally unable to operate in the style expected, or worse, if that department head is not measuring up in the actual performance of his duties, the administrator is forced either to let that person go or to shake up the authority structure. If the administrator is interested in learning what is going on down the line, and cannot, because of higher level blocks, he must go directly to the sources of information. When he has no confidence in his subordinates, he becomes loose. When he is satisfied they are performing satisfactorily along directions laid down by policy, he may be seen by some as being tight. But, *tight* is probably a poor word here. He wishes to leave to their own devices associates who are doing a good job, making himself available for consultation, advice, and judgment as indicated. The relationship can be still much more fraternal than authoritarian.

The good administrator, it seems to me, can mix it up, using whatever techniques are most appropriate to his immediate problems and his long-term goals. Rigidity of any type and a fixed status along such a continuum as the tight-loose continuum could be inimical to organizational interests. Furthermore, the conscientious administrator must progressively add to his repertoire of techniques useful in accomplishing purposes.

But no matter what the administrative style, the ways to fail and the ways to succeed are many. In a sense it is man against the system, man winning over the system or the system winning over man, and man using the system to accomplish its traditional goals. To lose, one need only to get tired, depressed, fed up, frustrated, defeated by accumulated irritations. Or one can run out of ideas, resources, creative solutions.

At such moments, one should remember the words of Theodore Roosevelt:

It is not the critic who counts, not the man who points out how the strong man stumbles, or where the doer of deeds could have done them better. The credit belongs to the man who is actually in the arena, whose face is marred by dust and sweat and blood, who strives violently, who errs and comes short again and again, who knows the great enthusiasm, the great devotion and spends himself in a worthy cause, who at the best knows in the end the triumph of high achievement, and who at the worst if he fails at least fails while daring greatly so that his place shall never be with those cold and timid souls who know neither victory nor defeat.

My thesis is that the odds are not so great that a vigorous administrator cannot emerge triumphant; that he has enormous implied resources if he will recognize and use them; that the times favor the forward movement of the state psychiatric hospital programs in concert with other developments; that, with proper management, the state hospital can evolve into a comprehensive health center (indeed, it is admirably situated in many instances to take leadership in this trend); that citizens are more interested than ever before in their human services system, including their state mental hospitals; that the job of leading such an organization can be exciting, growth-engendering, and immensely rewarding to patients, staff, and administrator alike.

REFERENCE

1. "Management Succession and Administrative Style," *Psychiatry* 30 (1967): 237–48.

Bibliography

Arsenian, J., and Semrad, E. V. " 'Depth' Levels in Individual Group Manifestations." *International Journal of Group Psychotherapy* 27 (1967): 82–97.

Barnard, C. I. *The Functions of the Executive.* Cambridge, Mass.: Harvard University Press, 1938.

Becker, A., ed. *The General Practitioner's Role in the Treatment of Emotional Illness.* Springfield, Ill.: Charles C Thomas, 1968.

Belknap, I. *Human Problems of a State Mental Hospital.* New York: McGraw-Hill, 1956.

Bellak, L. "Comprehensive Community Psychiatry Program at City Hospital." In *Handbook of Community Psychiatry and Community Mental Health,* ed. L. Bellak. New York: Grune and Stratton, 1964.

Berkind, H. "Psychiatric Inpatient Treatment of Adolescents: A Review of Clinical Experience. *Comprehensive Psychiatry* 3 (1962): 354–69.

Bonn, E., and Kraft, A. "The Fort Logan Mental Health Center: Genesis and Development." *Journal of Fort Logan Mental Health Center* 1 (1963): 17–27.

Caudill, W. *The Psychiatric Hospital as a Small Society.* Cambridge, Mass.: Harvard University Press, 1958.

Chien, Ching-piao. "Some Factors Deciding the Discharge of Chronic Mental Patients." *Hospital and Community Psychiatry,* (in press).

Clausen, J. A. "The Sociology of Mental Illness." In *Sociology Today,* ed. R. K. Merton, L. S. Broom, and L. Cottrell, pp. 485–508. New York: Basic Books, 1959.

Cohen, Melvin. "Work, as a Therapeutic Tool in the State Mental Hospital." *Mental Hygiene* 49, no. 3 (July 1965): 358–63.

Collins, Jerome. "Patient Helping Patient." *Hospital and Community Psychiatry* 18 (1967): 239–42.

Coplon, F. "The First Twenty-Four Hours at Boston State Hospital." Unpublished data.

Deutsch, A. *The Mentally Ill in America*. 2nd ed. New York: Columbia University Press, 1949.

DiMascio, A., and Levine, J. M. "A Step Toward Prediction of Clinical Efficacy: Relationship of History and Initial Characteristics of Patient to Improvement." In *Drug and Social Therapy in Chronic Schizophrenia*, ed. M. Greenblatt, M. Solomon, A. Evans, and G. Brooks. Springfield, Ill.: Charles C Thomas, 1965.

DiMascio, A., and Shader, R. I., eds. *A Handbook of Clinical Psychopharmacology*. New York: Science House, 1970.

Dohan, J. L. "Development of a Student Volunteer Program in a State Mental Hospital." In *The Patient and the Mental Hospital*, ed. M. Greenblatt, D. J. Levinson, and R. H. Williams, pp. 593–603. Glencoe: Free Press, 1957.

Duhl, F. J. "A Personal History of Politics and Programs in Psychiatric Training." Unpublished manuscript.

Ewalt, P. L., ed. *Mental Health Volunteers: The Expanding Role of the Volunteer in Hospital and Community Mental Health Services*. Springfield, Ill.: Charles C Thomas, 1966.

Expert Committee on Mental Health. Third Report. World Health Organization, Technical Report Series no. 73. Geneva: World Health Organization, 1953.

Gallagher, E. B.; Levinson, D. J.; and Erlich, I. "Some Socio-psychological Characteristics of Patients and Their Relevance for Psychiatric Treatment." In *The Patient and the Mental Hospital*, ed. M. Greenblatt, D. J. Levinson, and R. H. Williams, pp. 357–79. Glencoe: Free Press, 1957.

Garcia, L. B. "The Clarinda Plan: An Ecological Approach to Hospital Organization." *Mental Hospitals* 11 (1960): 30–31.

Gay, F. P. *The Open Mind: Elmer Ernest Southard*. Chicago: Normandie House, 1938.

Gelineau, V. A. "Explorations of the Volunteer Role: The Case Aide Program at Boston State Hospital." In *Mental Hospital Volunteers: The Expanding Role of the Volunteer in Hospital and Community Mental Health Services*, ed. P. L. Ewalt, pp. 35–44. Springfield, Ill.: Charles C Thomas, 1966.

Gelineau, V. A., and Evans, A. "Volunteer Case Aides Rehabilitate Chronic Patients." *Hospital and Community Psychiatry* 21 (1970): 90–93.

Gilbert, D. C., and Levinson, D. J. " 'Custodialism' and 'Humanism' in Mental Hospital Structure and in Staff Ideology." In *The Patient and the Mental Hospital,* ed. M. Greenblatt, D. J. Levinson, and R. H. Williams, pp. 20–35. Glencoe: Free Press, 1957.

Glasser, B. A. "Parental Attitudes Toward the Hospital Experience." In *Adolescents in a Mental Hospital,* ed. E. Hartmann, B. A. Glasser, M. Greenblatt, M. H. Solomon, and D. J. Levinson, pp. 82–89. New York: Grune and Stratton, 1968.

Glasser, B. A.; Hartmann, E. L.; and Avery, N. C. "Attitudes Toward Adolescents on Adult Wards of a Mental Hospital." *American Journal of Psychiatry* 124 (1967): 317–22.

Goffman, E. *Asylums.* New York: Doubleday–Anchor, 1961.

Greenblatt, M.; Emery, P. E.; and Glueck, B. C., Jr., eds. *Poverty and Mental Health.* Psychiatric Research Report 21. Washington: American Psychiatric Association, 1967.

Greenblatt, M.; Levinson, D. J.; and Williams, R. H., eds. *The Patient and the Mental Hospital.* Glencoe: Free Press, 1957.

Greenblatt, M.; York, R.; and Brown, E. L., eds. *From Custodial to Therapeutic Care in a Mental Hospital.* New York: Russell Sage Foundation, 1955.

Harrington, Michael. *The Other America.* New York: Macmillan, 1962.

Hartmann, E. *The Biology of Dreaming.* Springfield, Ill.: Charles C Thomas, 1967.

Hartmann, E.; Glasser, B. A.; Greenblatt, M.; Solomon, M. H.; and Levinson, D. J., eds. *Adolescents in a Mental Hospital.* New York: Grune and Stratton, 1968.

Henry, Jules, "Types of Institutional Structure." In *The Patient and the Mental Hospital,* ed. M. Greenblatt, D. J. Levinson, and R. H. Williams, pp. 73–90. Glencoe: Free Press, 1957.

Hodgson, R. C.; Levinson, D. J.; and Zaleznik, A. *The Executive Role Constellation.* Cambridge, Mass.: Division of Research, Harvard Business School, 1965.

Hollingshead, A. B., and Redlich, F. C. *Social Class and Mental Illness.* New York: John Wiley and Sons, 1958.

Jackson, G. W., and Smith, F. V. "A Proposal for Mental Hospital Reorganization: The Kansas Plan." *Mental Hospitals* 12 (1967): 5–8.

Joint Commission on Mental Illness and Health. *Action for Mental Health.* Final Report of the Commission. New York: Basic Books, 1961.

Jones, M. *The Therapeutic Community.* New York: Basic Books, 1963.

Kantor, D., and Gelineau, V. A. "Making Chronic Schizophrenics." *Mental Hygiene* 53, no. 1 (January 1969): 54–66.

Kotin, J., and Sharaf, M. R. "Intrastaff Controversy at a State Mental

Hospital: An Analysis of Ideological Issues." *Psychiatry* 30 (1967): 16–29.

————. "Management Succession and Administrative Style." *Psychiatry* 30 (1967): 237–48.

Kotin, J., and Schur, J. M. "Attitudes of Discharged Mental Patients Toward Their Hospital Experiences." *Journal of Nervous and Mental Disorders* 149 (1969): 408–14.

Kris, A. O., and Schiff, L. F. "An Adolescent Consultation Service in a State Mental Hospital: Maintaining Treatment Motivation." *Seminars in Psychiatry* 1 (1969): 15–23.

Kraus, E. A. *Pathways Back to the Community*. New York: Springer-Verlag, 1970.

Linn, L. "Some Aspects of a Psychiatric Program in a Voluntary General Hospital." In *Handbook of Community Psychiatry and Community Mental Health*, ed. L. Bellak. New York: Grune and Stratton, 1964.

McLardy, T. "Thalamic Microneurones." *Nature* 199 (1963): 820–21.

————. "Fornix Function During Behavior-Formative Age. *Scientific Proceedings of the American Psychiatric Association* 124 (1968): 42–43.

Miller, S. M., and Mishler, E. G. "Social Class, Mental Illness, and American Psychiatry: An Expository Review." *Milbank Memorial Fund Quarterly* 37 (1959): 174–99.

Minuchin, S. *Families of the Slums*. New York: Basic Books, 1967.

Myerson, D. J., and Mayer, J. "The Drug Addicts." In *The Practice of Community Mental Health*, ed. H. Grunebaum, pp. 197–218. Boston: Little, Brown, 1970.

Schoenfeld, T. Unpublished data on PROP, 1965.

Schulberg, H. C., and Baker, F. "The Changing Mental Hospital: A Progress Report." *Hospital and Community Psychiatry* 20 (1969): 159–65.

Schulberg, H. C.; Baker, F.; Notman, R.; and Bookin, E. "Treatment Services at a Mental Hospital in Transition." *American Journal of Psychiatry* 124 (1967): 506–13.

Sharaf, M. R., and Greenblatt, M. "Attitudes of Psychiatric Residents Toward Milieu Therapy." *Social Psychiatry* 9 (1968): 142–56.

Sharaf, M., and Levinson, D. J. "Patterns of Ideology and Role Definition Among Psychiatric Residents." In *The Patient and the Mental Hospital*, ed. M. Greenblatt; D. J. Levinson; and R. H. Williams, pp. 263–85. Glencoe: Free Press, 1957.

Srole, L.; Langer, T. S.; Michael, S. T.; Opler, M. K.; and Rennie, T. A. C. *Mental Health in the Metropolis*. New York: McGraw-Hill, 1961.

Stanton, A., and Schwartz, M. *The Mental Hospital*. New York: Basic Books, 1954.

Stotsky, B. *The Elderly Patient: Mental Patients in Nursing Homes*. New York: Grune and Stratton, 1968.

Ward, M. J. *The Snake Pit*. New York: Random House, 1946.

Weiner, L. "Developing a Consultation Program for Primary Physicians at a State Hospital." *Frontiers of Hospital Psychiatry*, Roche Report 5. no. 3. February 1968.

Weiner, L.; Becker, A.; and Friedman, T. T., eds. *Home Treatment: Spearhead of Community Psychiatry*. Pittsburgh: University of Pittsburgh Press, 1967.

Wilmer, H. A. "Toward a Definition of a Therapeutic Community." *American Journal of Psychiatry* 114 (1958): 824–34.

Index